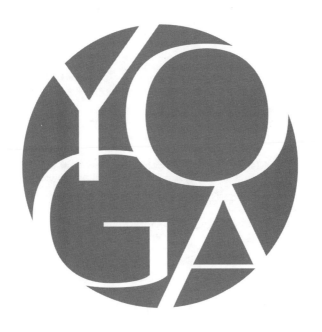

Some of the postures contained in this publication should only be attempted under the supervision of an experienced yoga practitioner. If in doubt, please contact your doctor or local yoga center.

Published by:
Ulysses Press
P.O. Box 3440
Berkeley CA 94703
www.ulyssespress.com

Library of Congress Control Number 2003104405
ISBN 1-56975-365-2

First published by HarperCollins Publishers, Sydney, Australia, in 2002.
This edition published by arrangement with HarperCollins Publishers Pty Ltd.

Printed in Canada by Transcontinental Printing

1 3 5 7 9 10 8 6 4 2

Cover: Kapotasana doubles pose
All photographs by Dhyan

Yoga models: Michael Asange, Jessie Chapman, Jamahl Chlopicki-Stocker, Kai Dennis, Fin Ellis, Lucy Roberts, Louisa Sear, Peter Watkins

YOGA
for
PARTNERS

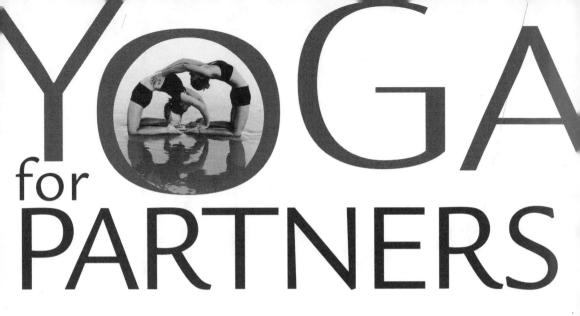

Over 75 Postures to Do Together

JESSIE CHAPMAN
PHOTOGRAPHS BY DHYAN

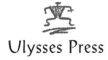

Ulysses Press

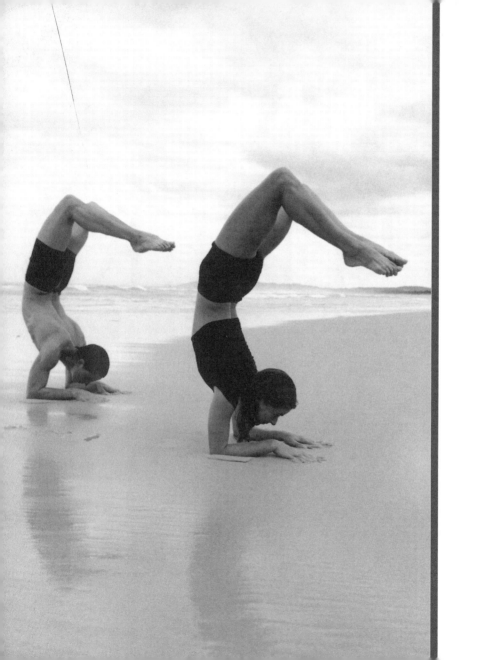

Contents

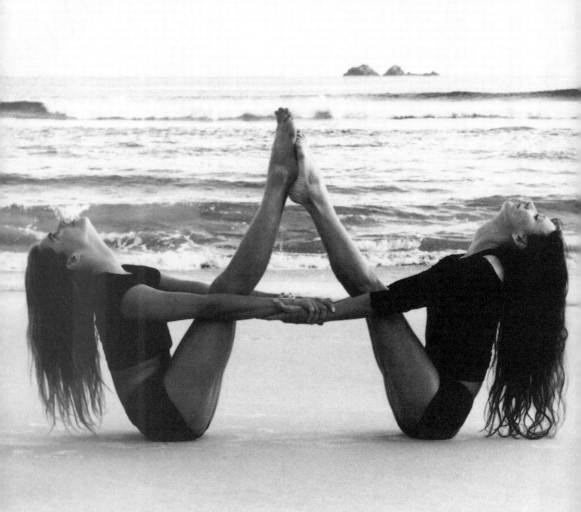

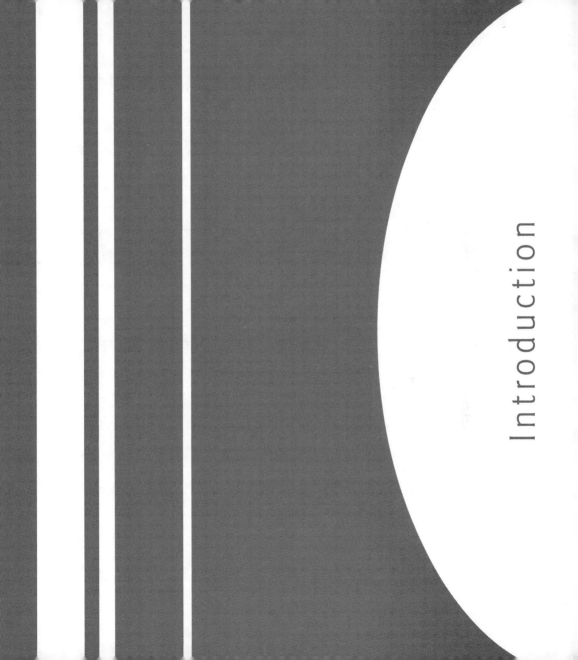

Introduction

A shared practice

Uniting in posture with a friend, lover or someone you have just met deepens our understanding of yoga and our awareness of others. Yoga is a form of bonding with the self and the world. Yoga-ing with a partner—breathing together, guiding and supporting one another—is a creative and playful journey that connects us to each other in the present moment.

Choosing to integrate yoga into our lifestyle often requires willpower, and having friends to practice with gives us the motivation to stick with it. With so many creative and intricate postures to explore, and so much to be gained and learned, partner yoga offers an inspiring way to encourage health and well-being to flourish in our life.

Derived from the Sanskrit word "yuj," yoga means union. Joining with a partner in practice reminds us that we live in a shared world. When we work together in a lighthearted space, beliefs and feelings of separation are replaced with a sense of belonging. As we learn about each other's differences, we discover our inherent similarities.

Just as regular yoga practice enriches one's sense of physical well-being, and mental and emotional health, partner yoga enhances our awareness of and sensitivity to others and brings new depth to our relationships. As in all relationships, there may be times of frustration and fear or joy and bonding. Being present with your partner throughout the practice and being aware of yourself and each other, are the keys to living spiritedly.

Yoga union

When we share *Asana* practice, we explore an intimate tradition that has been handed down from guru to disciple for thousands of years. This book is based on the physical postures. *Asana* literally means to be in posture with thoughts of the higher self, the divine or God in mind.

Holding in yoga postures, we learn to link the mind's intention with the body's movements and the breath. Coordinating with a partner adds another challenge, which develops awareness of our union.

Yoga's origins lie in ancient India and date back thousands of years. The many different disciplines of yoga practice all contribute to a holistic way of life and involve the practice of correct breathing and concentration, and the development of balance, coordination and focus.

Some key practices in yoga are *Asana* (physical postures), *Pranayama* (regulated breathing techniques), *Dharana* (concentration) and *Dhyana* (meditation), all of which lead to the ultimate goal of yoga's spiritual path—self-realization and the union of the self with all that is. Step into this sacred space together, where there is no separation.

Coming together

People are increasingly searching for deeper meaning in their lives and more intimacy with others. When we unlock our body in *Asana*, we often set free deeply stored emotions and feelings, which might not always feel comfortable. Being accepting of our self and each other and where we are at, and communicating openly with each other about what comes up, helps release and overcome negative emotions.

There may be times when you're feeling restricted by your partner's physical limitations or frustrated by your own. Overcome the need to strive, push or compete and allow for a practice in a space of sharing.

Yoga practice is a tool for gaining the confidence to overcome limiting lifestyle patterns, beliefs and fears that may be inhibiting our openness and closeness with others and our ability to live the life we want. To be together in practice is to revere each other's higher self and encourage each other to live life to our full potential.

Getting in touch

Human touch has proven healing powers. Children given lots of physical affection at birth are more likely to develop into confident and happy adults than children given little or no physical contact. We all have the ability to heal through touch, and when practicing yoga with a friend or lover we can assist them with their practice by simply placing a hand on their back for support or guidance. It can be the touch that helps keep them in the posture for longer, with more focus, dedication and understanding.

Whether practicing with your partner in a silent space or sharing advice, swapping ideas and learning from each other's personal experiences, yoga in union with others creates an atmosphere of growing and awakening. When you embrace yoga with a friend you motivate each other and encourage deeper connections and intimacy.

In addition, one's innate teaching skills are developed, as well as intuition and understanding.

United in breath

When making an adjustment to your partner's posture, unite the rhythm of your breathing with theirs for smooth, safe movements. As your partner inhales, inhale with them. As they exhale, exhale with them. Always breathe through the nose and follow the breathing instructions given in the posture.

If assisting your partner to lengthen or extend in a posture, work together with the breath. On the exhalation breath, the person being adjusted lets go and softens the muscles being opened, while the adjuster applies gentle pressure to encourage opening.

Remind your partner to deepen and lengthen their breathing, releasing any tension in the body with each exhalation breath. Sometimes it helps to close your eyes and to turn the awareness inward. Visualize tight muscles opening and tension melting away.

Communication & cooperation

We need to communicate clearly with each other in order to practice with awareness, and so we develop our communication skills. We become more sensitive to each other and are more able to assist each other to find a point of balance within.

Clear communication between partners improves the experience and understanding of the posture and increases the benefits of the pose. Start an adjustment by "checking in" with your partner. Ask whether they have practiced the posture before, if they've been adjusted in the pose before, and how their body feels.

Some days we may feel open in a particular posture, while other days we may feel more restricted. Encourage your partner to become aware of themselves, to listen to their own body and how it feels at that moment. When giving adjustments, remind your partner to let you know if something doesn't feel "right," and adapt the pose to suit.

The art of balance

You will soon discover how tricky it can be to do some of the *asanas* together. As you lean against each other in certain standing postures, it is easy to knock each other off balance. If you and your partner are different sizes, are at varying levels of flexibility or have different body shapes, a certain amount of focus will be required to work together effectively and with balance.

Sensitivity, a sense of humor and clear expression are the keys to partner yoga, as well as a sense of trust, which develops with practice. Some of the partner yoga postures included in this book are quite challenging and others very simple. Start with postures you feel comfortable with and begin to work on the more complicated ones when you and your partner feel ready.

Experiment and play with the postures, let your body and your intuition guide you to create postures that work for you and your partner. With practice your natural ability to create will emerge, and talents and skills such as balance, focus, strength, flexibility and understanding will develop.

Safe adjustments

Be sensitive when adjusting. Adjust with care and focus. Ask whether the pressure or adjustment is too strong or not strong enough. Don't push your partner into the perfect alignment or position, let them work sensitively with their breath and simply guide them into correct alignment and offer support and strength when required.

When breathing in unison with your partner and adjusting them into a deeper opening or extension, you can usually feel the points at which they let go. Their body releases tension and they extend further or deeper. At these points, you can apply gentle pressure to assist the opening already occurring, but always ask your partner if the adjustment feels okay.

If your partner wants a strong adjustment, build up to it with deep, slow breathing, allowing their body to release in its own time. This way you can assist your partner while avoiding the risk of strain, soft-tissue tears or other injuries.

You may be at a different level of practice than your partner but as long as you know yoga and are responsible for yourself, you'll benefit from (and enjoy) the postures in this book.

Basic guidelines

Practice: It is best to practice first thing in the morning when the stomach is empty, the mind peaceful and the external world quiet. However, as we all have different schedules and lifestyles, any time put aside to connect with yourself in yoga is the right time, morning, afternoon or evening.

Lightness: Yoga is best practiced on an empty stomach. If this is not possible, allow at least two hours after eating before practice, when the stomach is light.

Clothing: Wear loose, comfortable clothing made of natural, non-synthetic fibers, to ensure your skin can breathe. Don't wear shoes or socks so that you are in maximum contact with the ground.

Focus: To ensure a focused practice, find a quiet place away from any possible distractions. Take the phone off the hook, tell your family or housemates you're not to be disturbed, and be with your partner totally.

Space: Practice is best in a warm, dry environment out of direct sunlight and wind. A flat surface is good for balance and to help achieve correct alignment.

Breathing: Always breathe through the nose. Practice deep, full, slow inhalation and exhalation breaths. Aim to make the inhalation time equal to the exhalation time. Follow the breathing instructions given with the postures.

Relaxation: Always complete a practice with at least 5–10 minutes in *Savasana* (see page 184) to ensure your nervous system calms and you're fully relaxed before "re-entering the world."

Safety: Be sensitive and listen to your body's needs. Avoid inverted postures if you are menstruating, and postures that are going to make you tired. If you're pregnant, consult a prenatal yoga teacher for postures specifically designed for the comfort of you and your baby. While the practice of yoga is beneficial to our health and well-being on many levels, if you have a known or suspected illness or disease, consult a medical professional before attempting the postures in this book, or an experienced remedial yoga teacher for postures designed specifically for your individual needs.

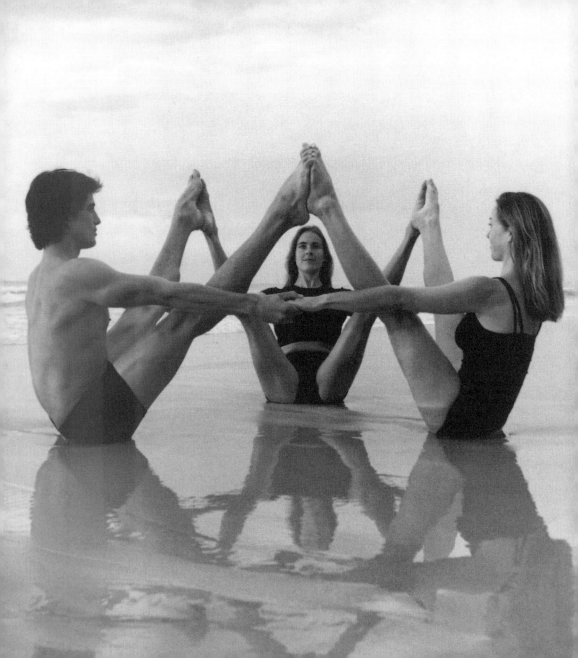

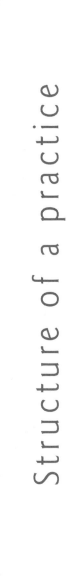

Structure of a practice

Creating a partner practice

The structure of a yoga practice varies according to an individual's needs, lifestyle and the time available. However, always begin by getting in touch with your breathing. Deep, full breathing, where the air moves into the lungs in an even, unrestricted flow, enables you to experience the benefits of yoga fully and promotes a relaxed, calm and balanced state of being.

Begin a partner session by connecting with each other. Choose one of the Beginning practices below; sit close to your partner and become aware of each other's breathing. Once a connection with your partner has been established, you're ready to begin. Decide which postures you'd like to practice: those that are beneficial for you both. Recognize where you are at, physically, mentally and emotionally on that day, and create a practice from that understanding.

Standing postures are good for developing strength and balance, and create a solid foundation to move from. Sitting postures develop flexibility and are good for targeting certain areas of the body; twisting poses are deeply cleansing and release built-up toxins; backward-bending postures release negative emotions and keep the body young; inverted postures stimulate the brain and re-energize; balancing postures promote focus and willpower; and relaxation postures relax!

When structuring a practice, ensure you're both sufficiently warmed up to prevent soft-tissue tearing, always allow time to wind a practice down with some relaxation postures and spend at least 5–10 minutes in *Savasana* (page 184). This way you'll feel centered after yoga. At the end of a practice, thank each other with the *Namaste* prayer (page 196), parting in a space of gratitude.

Beginning with the breath

Breathing is our common link with the sources of life and determines our state of being. How well we live depends greatly on how well we breathe. When we're stressed and anxious, we breathe short, shallow breaths, and when we're relaxed and calm, we breathe deep, full, unrestricted breaths.

Taking in a sufficient amount of oxygenated air is vital to our well-being physically, mentally, emotionally and spiritually. Relaxed breathing promotes a healthy circulatory system, providing the body with nutritious oxygenated blood and aiding in the elimination of wastes and the body's cleansing process.

The air we breathe contains *prana*, or life force. *Prana* is our life essence: the energy that links our physical self with essence, uniting our body and mind with our higher self. This *prana* gives us the vitality to live an inspired ("inspire" literally means to breathe in) and healthy life.

Always breathe in and out through your nose. When breathing, imagine the air moving through your body like a wave. First, the abdomen expands, then it contracts slightly as you draw the air up into your middle chest, expanding the ribs out to the sides. Then the whole chest expands and the collarbones lift slightly as the air reaches the top lobes of your lungs. Breathe fully so your lungs fill completely with air. As you exhale, draw your navel back to the spine slightly, expelling all the air from your lungs, feel your ribs contracting as the air leaves your body.

Moving with the breath

When in the postures, focus on the breath, using it as a tool; be in the postures in a relaxed yet energized manner. When we lose focus on the breath, it may become short and restricted, limiting the experience and benefits of the pose. As a general rule, lift and extend on the inhalation, and soften and let go on the exhalation.

When holding in a posture with a partner, synchronize your breathing. Inhaling and exhaling together, your two bodies become one. On the exhalation breath, soften together; on the inhalation breath, extend together. Your movements will become more united and harmonious, like a dance.

Styles of partner practice

Throughout this book you'll find three styles of partner yoga: Adjusting and Weightbearing, Doubles Yoga and Juxtapose. Experiment with all three types to create a practice that is inspiring for both partners.

ADJUSTING AND WEIGHTBEARING

While adjusting a partner in a pose, we learn to give pressure, touch and direction with sensitivity and effectiveness. The goal of adjusting is to bring your partner into correct alignment and to keep the spine lengthening and free from compression.

Through assisting we learn about the postures, how they affect different body types, and which postures are suitable for people with varying levels of flexibility.

Postures are sometimes performed more comfortably with the aid of a prop. These can vary from a chair or block to lean on, a blanket to rest on or a strap to lengthen with. When practicing with a partner, experiment with becoming a prop for each other.

Be inspired, adjust each other and explore the benefits of yoga for all. Yoga postures were, after all, developed by people like you and me, experimenting with themselves and others in postures.

DOUBLES YOGA

In Doubles Yoga two bodies come together and do the postures at the same time, creating intricate shapes. Balance and coordination are often required, along with a sense of humor! Each person must find a point of balance before merging with their partner in a pose without losing the connection within.

This can be a rather challenging way to practice. Compromise is often required to compensate for differing body types and heights, and clear communication is vital. Being in posture together can often make a practice stronger and deeper. When we have someone to lean against, we can go that little bit further in the space of trust.

JUXTAPOSE

Experiment with creating unique designs and inspiring symbols of unity. Yoga postures are incredibly intricate and creative, and when we juxtapose with someone they become even more beautiful.

Let your intuition be your guide and discover your inner yoga wisdom. Tune in to each other to create variations that reflect your collaboration with your partner.

Begin a partner practice by tuning in to each other with the breathing. Find a quite place to practice without distractions and center yourselves together in mind, body and spirit.

As we connect in yoga with the breath, our awareness is turned inward, away from thoughts of the past or future. This is a direct benefit of yoga, as the mind empties, the body relaxes and the whole being is refreshed. It's what brings people back to the practice time and time again.

Take a deep breath and let the united journey begin. From sitting or standing begin to lengthen and deepen your breathing, listening to the sound of your breath as you inhale and exhale in unison.

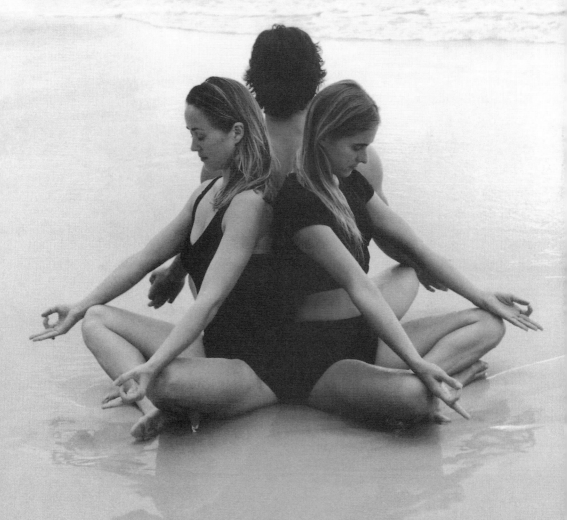

Tuning in

Back to back meditation

In the posture: Sit in a comfortable position, back to back with your partner. Your lower and upper backs meet. Sit up straight, lifting the lower part of your spine upwards. Roll your shoulders down and back to open your chest. Rest the back of your hands on your knees, palms facing upwards, close your eyes and tilt your forehead downward slightly.

Breathe: Inhale and exhale in unison. You may need to adjust your breathing to be in time with your partner. Aim for deep, full, even breathing through the nose.

Focus: Make the inhalation and exhalation last an equal length of time.

Practice: 25 smooth, even breaths through the nose.

Benefits: Establishes a connection with your partner through breath and touch; strengthens and elongates the spine and spinal muscles, opens the chest and shoulders, develops even breathing; calms the mind and cleanses the body.

Being present in the moment and with each other is a gift of yoga.

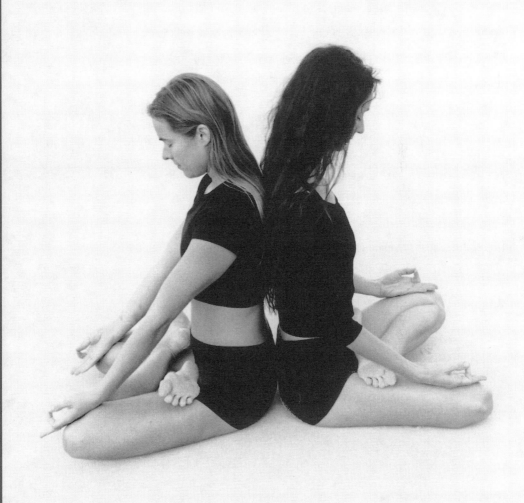

Peaceful reflections

In the posture: Sit in a comfortable position, facing your partner. Rest the back of your hands on your knees. Lift the lower part of your spine upwards. Roll your shoulders down and back, and breathe fully into your chest. Tuck your chin into your neck slightly and close your eyes.

Breathe: Inhale and exhale with slow, even breaths through the nose. Become aware of your partner's breathing rhythm and aim towards uniting yours with theirs.

Focus: Turn your gaze inward, remaining aware of your partner yet maintaining stillness within.

Practice: 25 slow, even breaths.

Benefits: Calms the mind and all the body's systems; develops a sense of togetherness and union; strengthens and elongates the spine.

Empty your mind and allow stillness to embrace you.

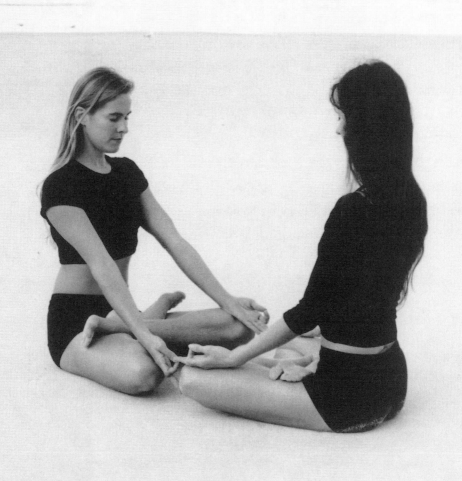

Back to back tadasana

In the posture: Stand back to back. Have the backs of your bodies touching. Tuck your buttocks under slightly, lengthen out from your hips and roll your shoulders down and back to open the chest. Extend your fingers and arms straight down at your sides, bringing your palms together. Have your head upright and face forward. Begin to breathe deep, full breaths, gradually lengthening the inhalations and exhalations. Once you feel centered together in *Tadasana*, begin to breathe in unison.

Breathe: Inhale and exhale fully.

Focus: On finding unity with your partner through synchronized breathing, keep your posture straight and your whole body activated.

Hold: 25 deep, full breaths or until you are both feeling centered.

Benefits: Connects you with your partner in preparation for the practice.

Find **yourself** and each **other** standing tall, **centered** and focused in **yoga**.

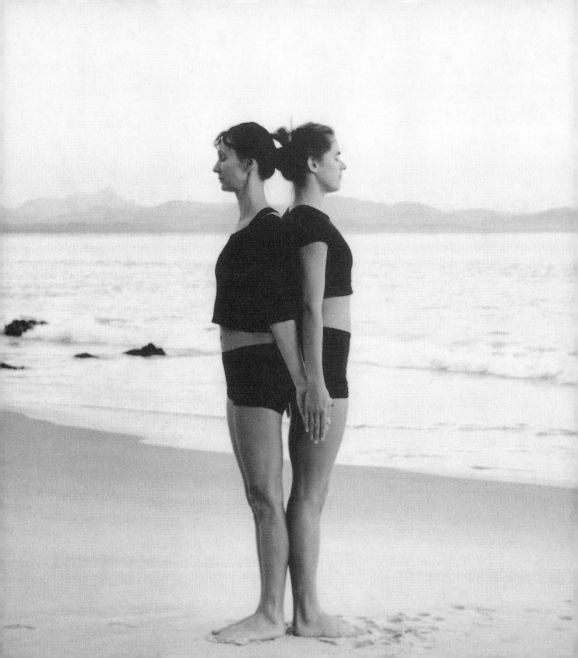

The dynamic standing postures develop strength and willpower. They build strong legs, feet and ankles, and develop a solid foundation on which to stand. With a stable base, our upper body moves more freely and gracefully. Correct posture is created through standing tall and lengthening the spine and limbs.

Practicing with a partner is motivating, and you are able to help each other position your bodies. A partner can check the alignment of your hips, see your legs are working strongly, adjust your feet, help lengthen your spine, encourage a twist, open the chest and shoulders, and point out where you need to soften and release tension. These simple adjustments can improve your practice and increase the benefits of a pose.

Develop your combined practice and build on it with confidence. Find out each other's physical weaknesses and strengths, and choose postures you both feel comfortable with. Being together in yoga develops awareness and sensitivity as you strive to unite in a posture with correct alignment. When practicing a standing posture back to back with a partner, balance is required. If the weight of your body is too much for your partner, they may lose their balance.

Avoid standing postures if you have high blood pressure, heart problems or nervous disorders; seek medical advice if you're unsure. Take extra care if you have knee or back problems, and avoid during the first trimester of pregnancy and the first few days of menstruation if your energy levels are low.

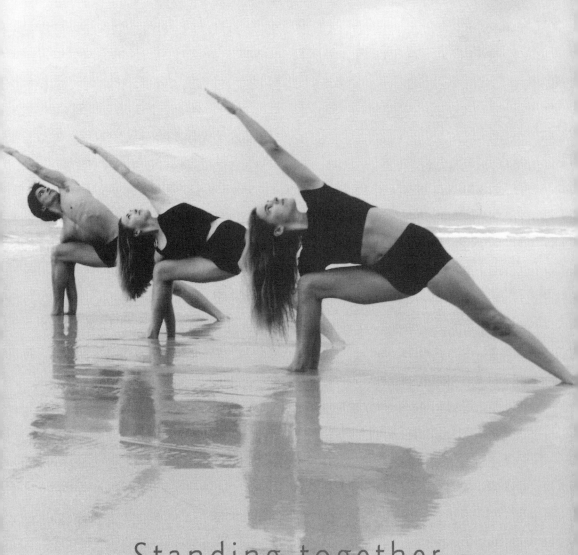

Standing together

Tadasana
connection sequence

TADA—MOUNTAIN

In the posture: Stand back to back with your partner, the palms of your hands touching. Spread your toes wide, activate your leg muscles, and draw your kneecaps and thighs upwards. Gently squeeze and tuck your buttocks under, and roll your shoulders down and back to open your chest. Visualize energy flowing upwards from the ground, through your legs, torso and out through the crown of your head.

Breathe: Begin by synchronizing your breathing with your partner's then start moving with the breath. On the inhalation, elevate your arms; on the exhalation, release them down. Keep your arms touching your partner's as you flow.

Focus: Keep the movement of your bodies flowing evenly with the breath.

Practice: 5–10 cycles, to tune into each other and the breath.

Benefits: Promotes deep, full breathing; opens the chest, heart and lungs; promotes correct posture and synchronization with your partner.

Link together in body, breath and intention; become one in a harmonious wave-like movement.

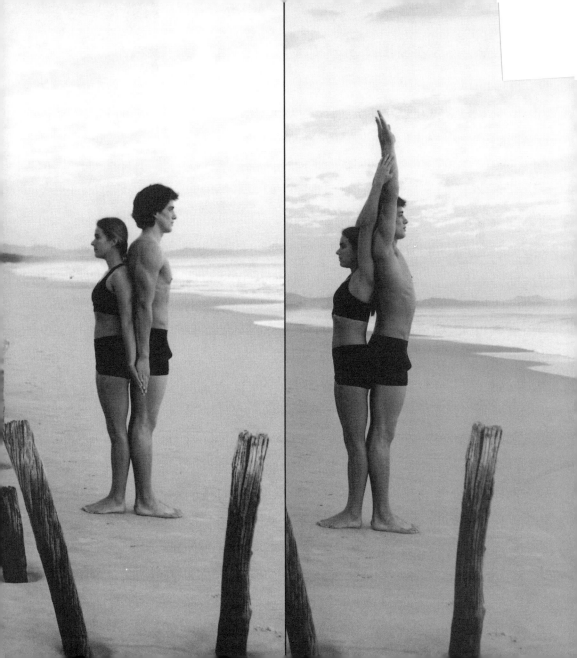

Vrksasana joining

VRKSA—TREE

In the posture: Stand beside your partner with your inside arms around each other's waist. Bend your outside leg, placing the foot up into your thigh. Bring your outside arm to the middle, joining palms in front at the center, becoming one being in balance and prayer. Find a point in front of you at eye level to gaze at, empty your mind of thoughts and be together in stillness.

Breathe: Inhale and exhale together in united breath.

Focus: Keep your standing leg locked; press your thigh into your foot and foot into your thigh. Maintain a soft gaze forward at eye level.

Hold: 5–10 breaths, then exhale to release the leg down and change sides.

Benefits: Creates a space of intimacy in quietness; stretches and flexes the knee and hip joints; develops balance and mental focus.

Merge together in a warm embrace—balanced beings in prayer and concentration.

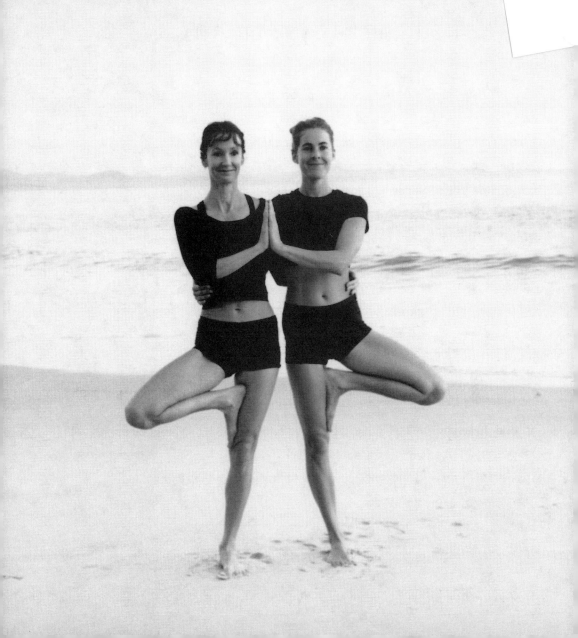

Trikonasana adjustment

TRIKONA–TRIANGLE

In the posture: One partner begins. Step your feet about four feet apart. Turn your left foot in 15° and your right foot out to a 90° angle. Activate your leg muscles, lift your kneecaps and thighs upwards. Extend your arms out at shoulder height. Inhale to stretch and lengthen the right arm and right side of the torso over to the right, exhale and place your hand onto your right foot, or wherever it reaches along your right leg. Tuck in your chin as you face upwards. Extend your left arm up to form a straight line with your right arm. Draw your shoulder blades in.

Adjuster: Stand behind your partner. Place your left hand on their left hip, your right hand on their left arm. Remind them to rotate their left hip back as you pull it with your hand. Draw their left arm up.

Breathe: Use soft breathing to stay relaxed and balanced in the pose.

Focus: Gaze beyond your left hand. Envision yourself in triangular alignment. Keep your leg muscles activated.

Hold: 5–10 full breaths, then release and change sides.

Variations: Place your right hand on a block if you have trouble reaching your leg. Keep your right leg bent for support if needed. Look down if looking upward strains your neck.

Benefits: Strengthens the legs, ankles and spinal muscles; tones the organs, and digestive and nervous systems; stretches the torso muscles.

Fine-tune your alignment to create a three-edged triangle—sharp, straight and strong.

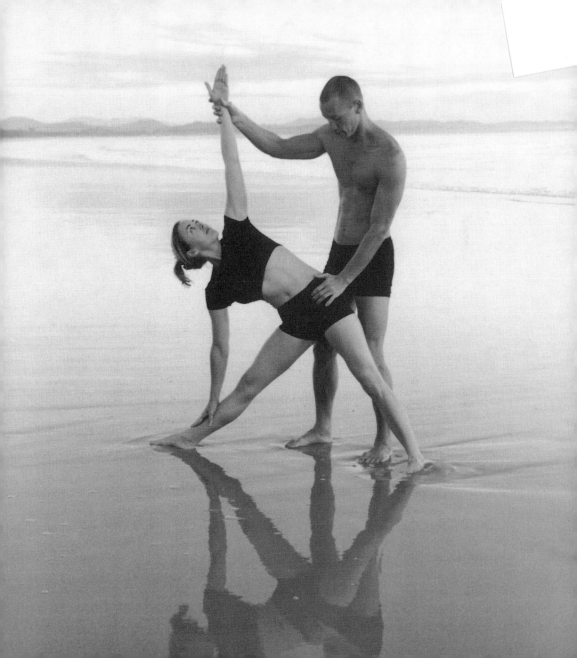

Trikonasana back to back

TRIKONA—TRIANGLE

In the posture: Stand back to back with your partner, your own feet about a yard apart. Turn your right foot out 90˚ and your left foot in 15˚. Inhale to lift out of the waist, extending your arms out at shoulder height. Exhale to lengthen and release over your right leg, placing your right hand onto your partner's left ankle behind you. Activate and contract your front leg muscles, drawing them upwards, and rotate your left hip back. Tuck your chin in and turn to look beyond your left hand. Keep your chin tucked in to protect your neck from straining.

Breathe: Take deep full breaths in time with your partner.

Focus: Open your left hip, strengthen your legs and rotate your chest upwards.

Hold: 5–10 deep full breaths, then release and change sides.

Variation: Look down at the floor if it strains your neck to look upwards.

Benefits: Tones the legs, developing a strong and balanced foundation for standing; lengthens the spine and tones the spinal muscles.

Find your **point** of **balance** then lean into each other to discover a **united** center.

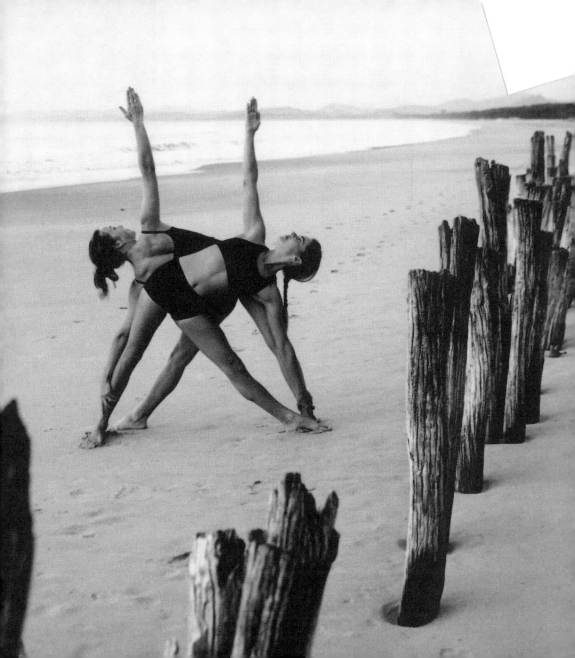

Padottanasana
shoulder release

PADA—FOOT/LEG; UTTAN—EXTENDED

In the posture: One partner begins in standing position, feet about a yard apart, heels turned out slightly so the outside edges of the feet are parallel. Contract and lift the shinbones, kneecaps and thighs. Interlock your fingers behind your back, bringing the heels of your hands together. Take a deep breath and on the exhalation bend at the hips, coming forward and down, releasing your arms over your head. Tuck your chin in and look to your navel. Bring your body weight towards the balls of your feet.

Adjuster: Stand beside your partner with your knees slightly bent and your left leg supporting their right leg. Place your left hand onto their lower back and your right hand onto their wrists. As your partner softens, move their hands toward the ground, allowing their shoulders to release. Make your adjustment gradual.

Breathe: Deep, full breaths and soften any tension on the exhalation.

Focus: Bringing the heels of the hands together.

Hold: 5–10 breaths, then release and swap positions with your partner.

Benefits: Releases stiff shoulders and arms; softens the back muscles; strengthens and stretches the legs; tones the abdominal organs and stimulates digestion.

Soften and release into the shoulders and feel them melting open with each out breath.

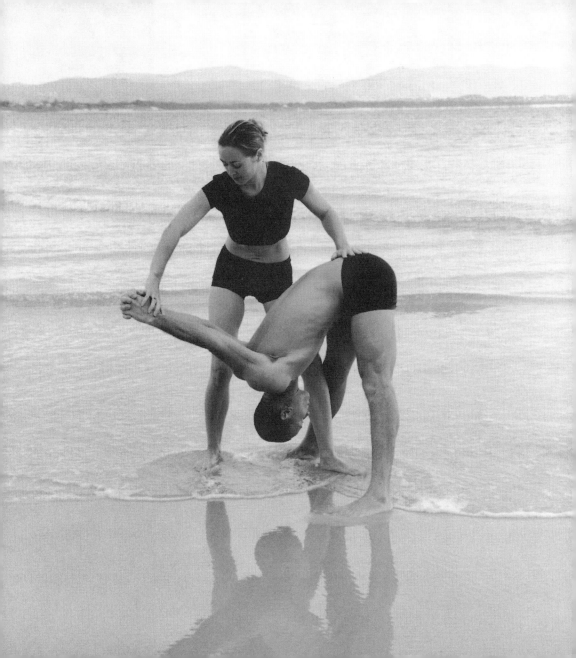

Padottanasana adjustment

PADA—FOOT/LEG: UTTAN—EXTENDED

In the posture: One partner begins in standing position, feet about a yard apart. Inhale to lift out of the waist and exhale to slowly bend at the hips and come forward and down. Place the palms of your hands between your feet on the floor, tuck your chin in and look to your navel. Let your head and neck be soft and draw your torso in toward the knees. Lift your shoulders back and away from your ears. Keep your kneecaps and thighs lifting, and move your body weight forward to the balls of your feet.

Adjuster: Stand beside your partner. Place one hand on their lower back and one hand on their upper back. With gentle pressure, encourage their spine to lengthen down and in toward their legs. Protect your own back by standing with your front leg bent and your back leg locked.

Breathe: Take deep, full breaths; exhale, releasing into the posture.

Focus: Soften the spine and relax the head, neck and facial muscles.

Hold: 5–10 breaths, then swap positions with your partner.

Variation: Keep your knees bent for support; place your hands on blocks for lift.

Benefits: Stretches and lengthens the muscles at the back of the legs; softens and loosens the back; stimulates blood flow to the brain.

Encourage **loosening** and elongation of your **partner's** spine with a firm **adjustment.**

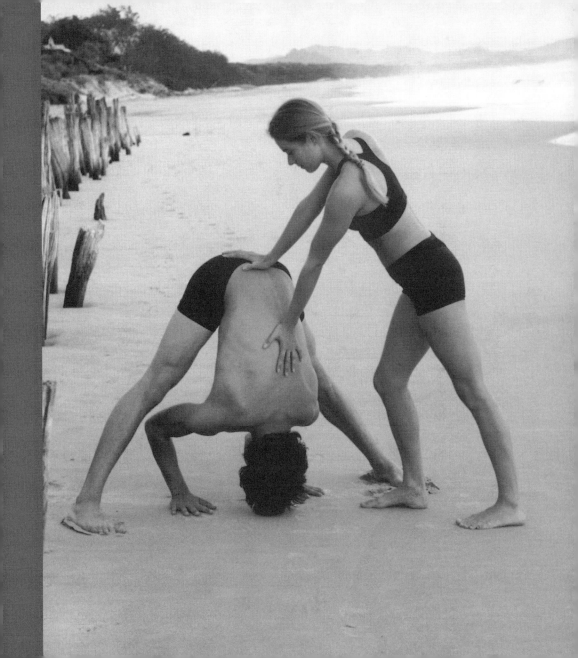

Padottanasana stretch

PADA—FOOT/LEG; UTTAN—EXTENDED

In the posture: Stand back to back with your partner, about a yard apart. Step your feet a yard apart with the outside edges parallel to each other. Inhale to lift out of your waist, exhale to soften and release forward and down. Keeping your legs locked, bring your arms through inside your legs to hold onto each other's forearms. Release deeper into the back-leg stretch as you move your hands further along your partner's arms, letting your spine release forward and down. Tuck your chin in and gaze up to your navel.

Breathe: Allow the breath to soften you into the pose; release any tension in the legs and spine.

Focus: Keep the spine extending and the legs locked.

Hold: 5–10 breaths, then release up slowly.

Benefits: Stretches the hamstring muscles; extends and releases the spine; increases blood flow to the brain and circulation to the upper body; relieves fatigue; develops coordination and focus, and promotes balance.

Finding steadiness within, draw toward each other for deep opening and elongation.

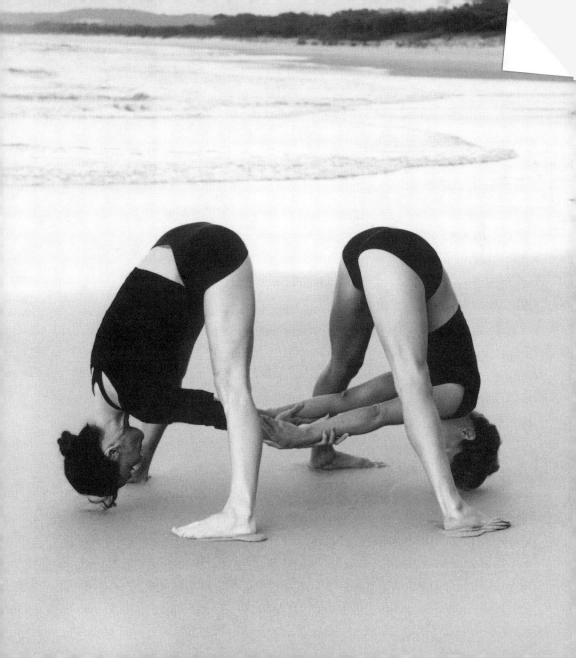

Padottanasana joining

PADA—FOOT/LEG; UTTAN—EXTENDED

In the posture: Stand back to back with your partner. On the exhalation breath, bend at the hips and hang forward so the back of your legs and buttocks are touching your partner's. When you have found a point of balance, slowly wrap your arms around your partner's shoulders. Do this one at a time. Lock your legs and draw in close to each other, softening your spine down and stretching the back of your legs.

Breathe: When in position, breathe in unison with your partner.

Focus: Maintain soft eye contact with each other and a center point of balance.

Hold: 5–10 deep, full breaths. To come up, release out of the pose one at a time.

Benefits: Stretches the hamstring muscles; extends and releases the spine; increases blood flow to the brain and circulation to the upper body; relieves fatigue; develops coordination and focus, and promotes balance.

Focus, coordination, balance and breath—key tools for uniting in yoga.

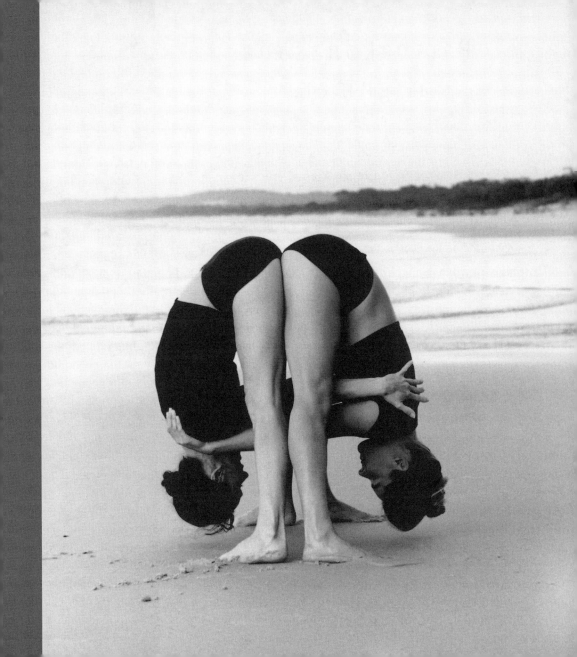

Parsvakonasana
alignment

PARSVA—SIDEWAYS: KONA—ANGLE

In the posture: One partner begins in standing position, feet about four feet apart. Turn your right foot out 90° and your left foot in 15°. Inhale and lift out of your waist, extending your arms away from each other. Exhale as you bend your right knee into a right angle, and place your right hand on the floor on the outside of your right foot. Inhale and extend your left arm over your head, keeping your buttocks activated and your leg muscles strong. Tuck your chin in and gaze back toward your left hand. Keep the underside of your bent leg lifted.

Adjuster: Stand behind your partner and check their alignment. Create one straight line from the little-toe side of their extended leg, out of their hip, shoulder, up their arm and out through the fingertips.

Breathe: Soft, calm breathing through the nose.

Focus: Create a straight line with the outside edge of your body.

Hold: 5–10 deep, full breaths, then release and swap positions.

Variation: Look down at the floor if it strains your neck to look upwards. Place your right hand on a block for extra support.

Benefits: Opens the hips; strengthens the legs and the soft tissue supporting the knee joint; stimulates the internal organs and nervous system; elongates the spinal muscles and vertebrae.

Straight-sided body creating one sharp line from the toes out through the fingertips.

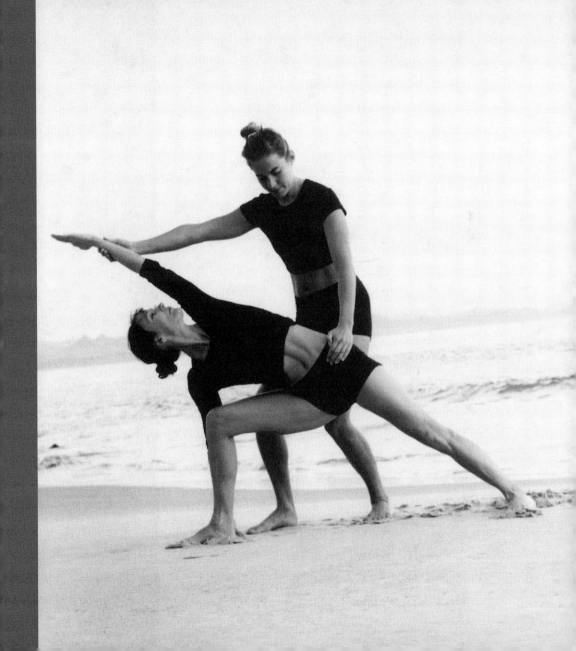

Virabhadrasana I
adjustment

VIRA—WARRIOR FROM INDIAN MYTHOLOGY

In the posture: One partner begins in standing position, feet about four feet apart. Turn your right foot out 90° and your left foot in 45°. Rotate your right hip back and your left hip forward so the hips are parallel. Inhale and lift out of your waist, extending your arms upwards. As you exhale, lunge downward to create a 90° angle with the right leg, your knee above the ankle. Lift and extend out of your hips, lengthening upwards. Focus forward or look up beyond your palms.

Adjuster: Stand beside your partner, assuming the same position as them. Place your hands on their hips and rotate their right hip back and left hip forward so they are parallel. Check that their back leg is straight and they are working into the little-toe side of their foot and lifting the underside of both legs.

Breathe: Inhale and exhale fully through the nose, expanding the chest.

Focus: Strengthen the base, feet and legs; extend upwards with the torso; activate the arms and lock the elbows.

Hold: 5 breaths, then release and change sides. Then swap positions with your partner.

Benefits: Strengthens the legs and knee joints; lengthens the spine and strengthens the spinal muscles; develops willpower.

Be in position to tone and vitalize the whole body, from the base up.

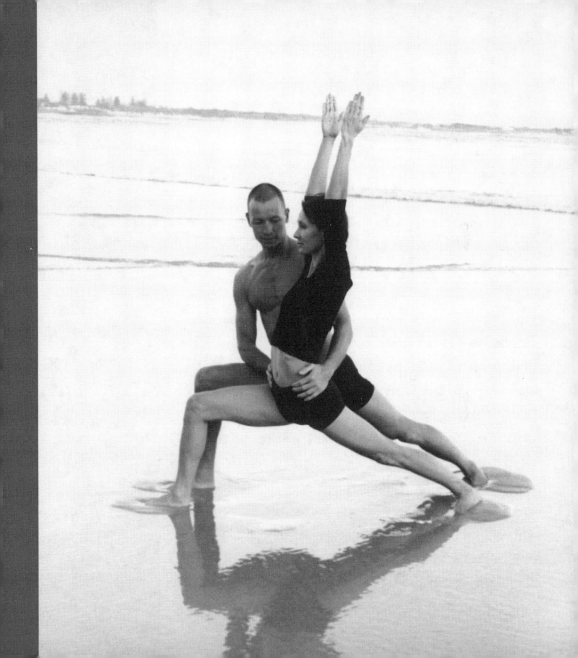

Virabhadrasana II adjustment

VIRA—WARRIOR FROM INDIAN MYTHOLOGY

In the posture: One partner begins in standing position, feet about four feet apart, right foot turned out 90° and left foot turned in 15°. Align the heel of your right foot with the inner arch of your left foot. As you inhale, extend your arms out to the side, and lengthen out from your waist. As you exhale, bend your right knee to a right angle, opening your right hip. Keep your left leg straight and locked. Squeeze your buttocks and lean your torso back slightly over your back leg so your torso is centered above the pelvis. Turn your head to face the right and extend your arms away from each other.

Adjuster: Stand beside your partner, and assume the same position. Rotate their left hip back. Check that their back leg is straight.

Breathe: Take deep breaths, expanding the chest on inhalation.

Focus: Keep your pelvic floor muscles lifted, legs activated and torso extending upwards.

Hold: 5–10 breaths, then release and change sides. Then swap positions with your partner.

Benefits: Strengthens the legs, and the knee and ankle joints; tones the spinal muscles and nervous system.

Precaution: Be careful if you have weak knee joints.

Stretch and strengthen into accurate position with your partner as a prop.

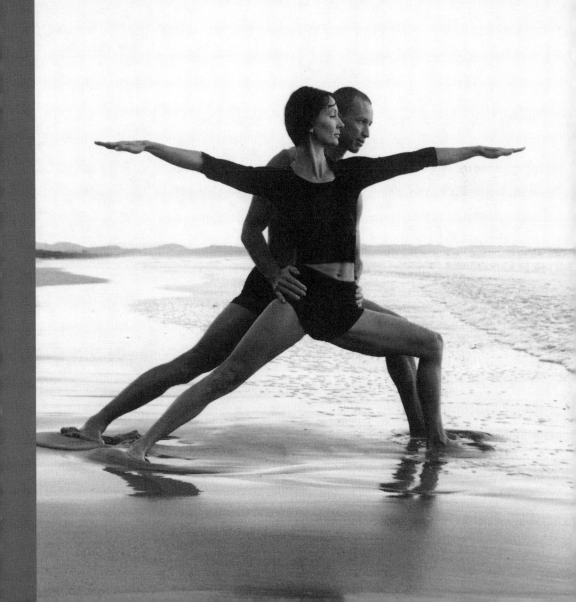

Virabhadrasana II joining

VIRA—WARRIOR FROM INDIAN MYTHOLOGY

In the posture: Begin by standing beside your partner at a yard's distance. Move into *Virabhadrasana II* in opposite directions, positioning your back leg so the outside edge of your back foot is touching your partner's and pressing into the ground. Bend your front leg to create a 90° angle. Open your hips so they are facing forward. Raise your arms and extend them away at shoulder height and lift your chest. Join your back hand with your partner's and turn to look over your forward hand. Keep your torso centered above your pelvis.

Breathe: Take deep, full inhalations and exhalations, softening in the pose with the breath.

Focus: Align yourself accurately in the posture and be in the pose without throwing your partner off balance. Keep lifting your chest.

Hold: 5–10 breaths, then release and repeat on the opposite side.

Benefits: Strengthening and toning posture for the whole body; particularly effective for developing strong legs and knee joints.

Two focused beings find strength and willpower in partner practice.

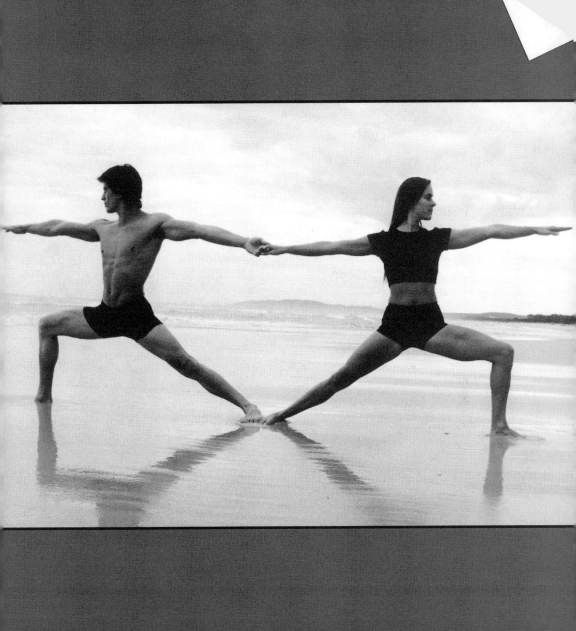

Virabhadrasana III
joining

VIRA—WARRIOR FROM INDIAN MYTHOLOGY

In the posture: One partner comes into the pose, balancing on their right leg first, the other on their left leg. Begin by standing facing each other about six and a half feet apart. Bend your front leg, and as you exhale lean forward over your bent leg. Moving your body weight forward, begin to raise your other leg off the ground as you straighten your front leg. Once you are balanced and both legs are locked, drop the hip of your raised leg so it is parallel to your standing-leg hip. Inhale and extend you arms forward to hold each other's shoulders, and look toward your partner. With the support of your partner, focus on keeping your hips even, back straight and both legs activated.

Breathe: Inhale and exhale in unison with your partner.

Focus: Stay lifted and balanced.

Hold: 5–10 even breaths, then release down gracefully and change legs.

Variation: If you are both finding the balancing position difficult, practice it one at a time, the other partner taking the weight of the person in the pose.

Benefits: Strengthens the legs, lower back and abdominals; improves balance and coordination; develops willpower as you hold the pose.

Reach out for your partner and find support and centering in each other.

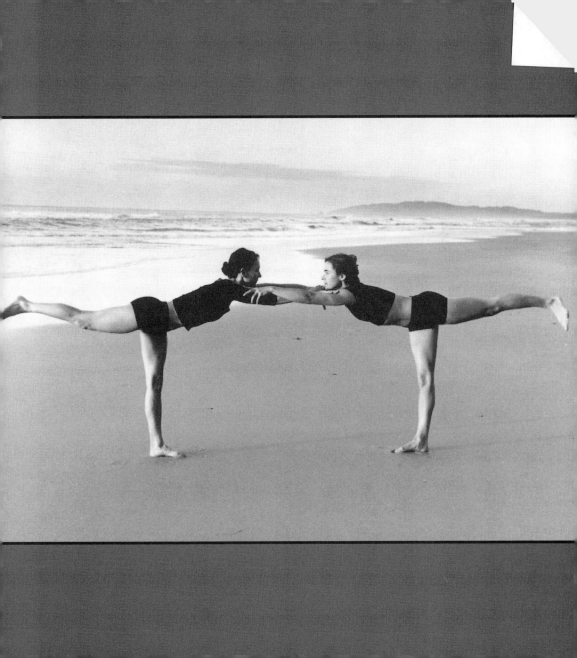

Ardha chandrasana adjustment

ARDHA—HALF; CHANDRA—MOON

In the posture: Begin with one partner standing with feet apart. Slowly lean over to your right side, bending your right leg and placing your right hand on the ground, about a foot in front of your right foot. As you straighten your right leg, raise your left leg off the ground and bring it to a straightened point, creating a right angle with the other leg. Roll your left hip back. Lift your left arm, straighten both arms, tuck your chin in and turn to look up beyond your left hand.

Adjuster: Once they are balanced, stand behind your partner and place your left hand on their left hip and your right hand on their left hand. Gently rotate the hip back to open it. Extend their left arm upward, keeping it aligned with their right arm.

Breathe: As you hold in the posture, focus on breathing in unison.

Focus: Keep your raised leg in line with your hip and legs locked.

Hold: 5–10 deep, full breaths, then release down and change legs.

Variation: Look forward or down at the ground if looking upward is straining your neck. Keep your legs bent if needed.

Benefits: Promotes balance and focus; strengthens and tones the leg muscles; strengthens the muscles of the knee joints and spine; opens the pelvic muscles.

A challenging **balancing** posture that encourages **flexibility** of body and mind.

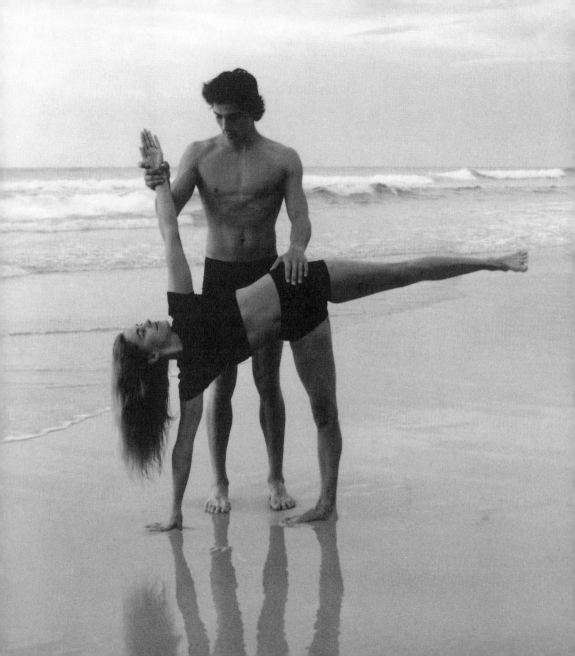

Seated on air

In the posture: This pose is normally practiced up against a wall, but in this case you become a wall of support for your partner and they for you. Stand with your feet hip-width apart and your back pressing against your partner's. As you exhale, bend your knees and release down, walking your feet out until your lower legs form a right angle with your upper legs, hips in line with your knees, and knees in line with your ankles. Tuck your tailbone under and press firmly into each other's back for support. Link arms for support, rest your hands on your knees, or try raising your arms above your head and joining hands.

Breathe: Inhale and exhale softly and evenly through the nose while maintaining the pose.

Focus: Strengthen the legs and stay seated.

Hold: 10 breaths or as long as is comfortable. To release, walk your feet in as you slide up to standing.

Benefits: Strengthens the muscles of the legs and knee joints; tones the back and abdominal muscles; develops focus and coordination.

Rest in **calm** as you sit in mid-air, relying on each other's **strength** and support for **balance**.

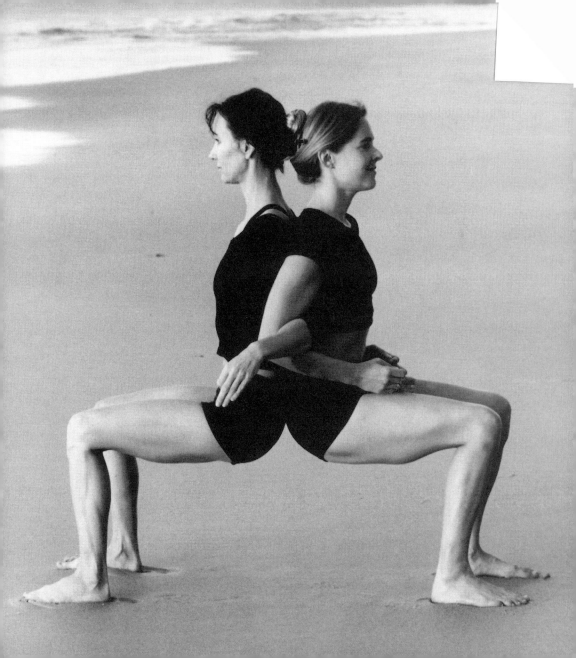

Parighasana at the hips

PARIGHA—GATE

In the posture: Both partners position into the pose, one leaning to the right and the other to the left. Kneel side by side with your inside hips touching. Extend your outside leg to the side, creating a straight line, and turn the foot in 45°. Place your outside hand onto your extended leg. Inhale, raising the inside arm and extending out of your waist. Exhale and extend your arm over your head, the palm facing down. Tuck in your chin and look beyond your raised arm.

Breathe: Inhale and exhale fully through your nose.

Focus: Extend out from the waist, elongate your spine and stretch the side of your torso.

Hold: 5–10 breaths, then release and change sides.

Variation: Turn your head to look downward if looking upward is straining your neck.

Benefits: Stretches and tones the lateral torso muscles, abdominal organs and muscles of the chest and arms; extends the spine and massages the spinal muscles and kidneys; tones the spinal nerves.

Joined at the hip, two bodies unite to lengthen out of the hips and away from each other.

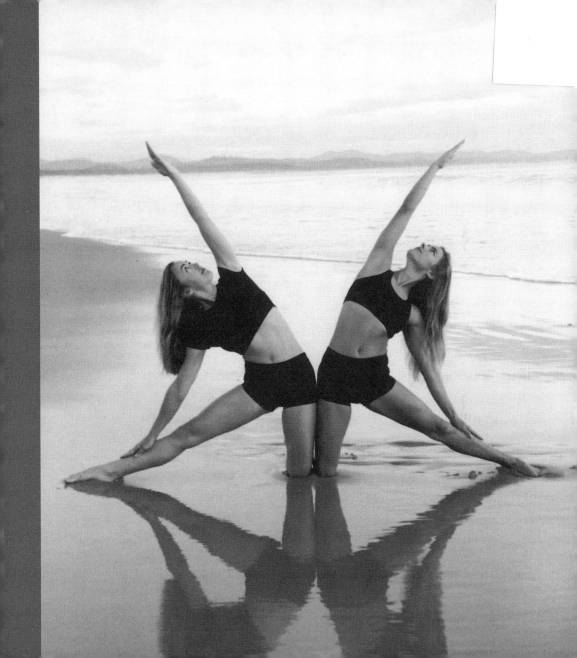

Parighasana at the toes

PARIGHA–GATE

In the posture: Both partners position into the pose, one leaning to the right and the other to the left. Kneel side by side and place your hands on your hips. Exhale and extend your inside leg toward your partner, keeping the foot in line with your hip, the toes of your extended leg touching your partner's. Place your inside arm on your leg down toward the foot. Inhale to raise your outside arm and extend out from your waist. Exhale and extend your arm over your head, the palm facing down. Tuck in your chin and look beyond your raised arm.

Breathe: Inhale and exhale together for synchronized releasing.

Focus: Release out of the outside hip, keeping it above the knee.

Hold: 5–10 breaths, then release up and change sides.

Variation: Look downward if looking upward is straining your neck. Try joining hands if you have the flexibility; if you cannot join hands, aim in that direction. Different body heights and levels of flexibility will vary the pose.

Benefits: Stretches and tones the lateral torso muscles, abdominal organs and muscles of the chest and arms; extends the spine and massages the spinal muscles and kidneys; tones the spinal nerves.

A stimulating lateral stretch to rejuvenate often untouched areas of the body.

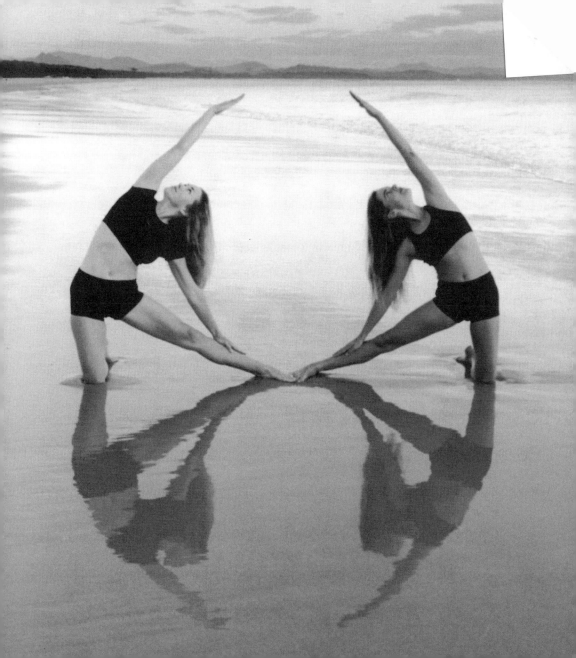

Parighasana opposite stretch

PARIGHA—GATE

In the posture: Kneel side by side with your partner. Extend your inside leg out to the side so the side of your foot touches your partner's. From here, place your outside hand on the floor beside your kneeling leg for support. Raise your inside arm up and extend it over your head. Create a straight, arrow-like line all the way from your toes to your fingertips. Tuck your chin in and turn to look beyond your fingertips. Aim to create a V-shaped line between the sideways extensions of you and your partner.

Breathe: Inhale and exhale evenly through your nose.

Focus: Lengthen out of your hip and extend the whole side of your body.

Hold: 5 breaths, then release and repeat on the other side.

Variation: Look to the floor if it is straining your neck to look upwards.

Benefits: Stretches the lateral torso muscles and the whole side of the body; strengthens the legs, arms and spinal muscles; develops willpower and focus.

Discover beauty and strength in two forms, extending and elongating sideways.

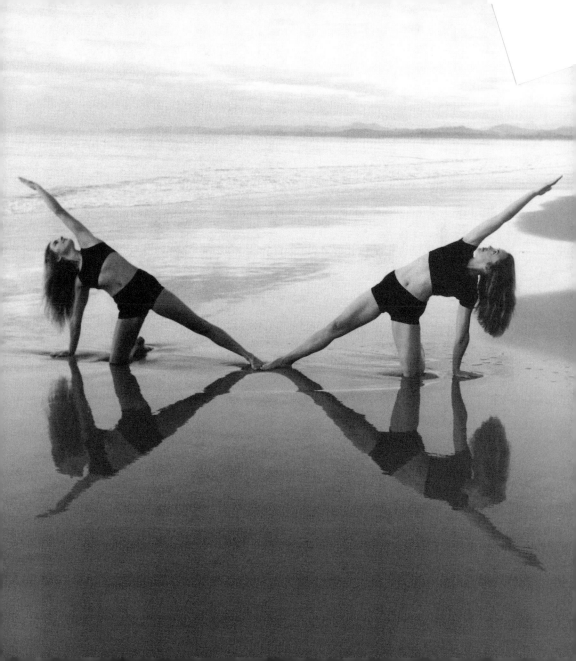

Uttanasana stretch

UTTANA–EXTENSION

In the posture: Stand back to back with your partner, about a yard apart, your feet hip-width apart. On the exhale, bend forward and down, moving your head toward your knees. Draw your kneecaps up and activate your thighs. Bring your arms around the outside of your legs to join your partner's, hold each other's wrists. Take your grip farther up their arm and pull toward your partner until you feel a deep opening in the back of your legs. Keep your chin tucked in and your spine lengthening down.

Breathe: Inhale to extend, exhale to soften and release.

Focus: Lengthen your spine.

Hold: 5–10 breaths or as long as is comfortable. Release slowly when ready.

Variation: If you are not able to bring your head all the way into your knees, work where you are with the breath and be sensitive to your partner.

Benefits: Stretches the hamstring muscles; elongates the spine; stimulates metabolism; increases blood flow and circulation to the brain.

Linked in a forward stretch, pulling inward for increased opening and revitalization.

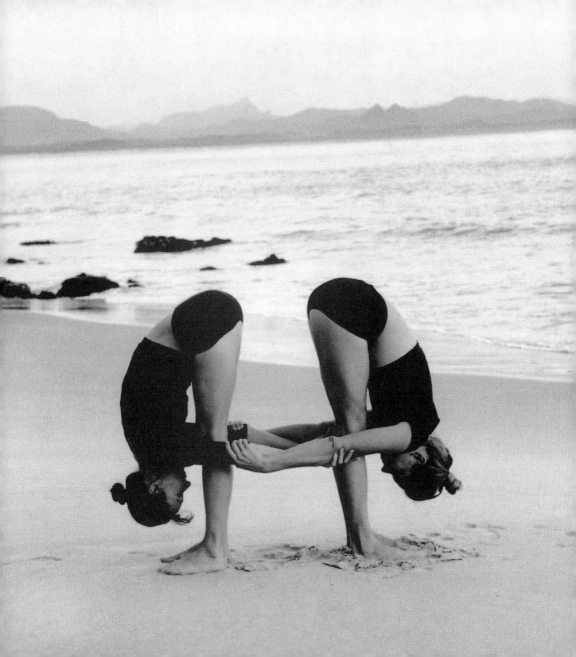

Uttanasana wrap

UTTANA–EXTENSION

In the posture: Stand back to back with your partner, your buttocks touching. Bend at the hips, and hang forward and down so you are looking at your partner through your legs. Place your hands in front of you for support and position your legs so they are touching your partner's. From here the challenge is to hold onto each other's ankles without toppling over. Get into the posture one at a time. The trick is not to lean too far forward or back, but to remain centered, so you don't unbalance your partner. If you accomplish this step, next try wrapping your arms around each other's shoulders.

Breathe: Inhale and exhale through the nose.

Focus: Maintain your point of balance.

Hold: 5–10 deep, slow breaths.

Benefits: Encourages a sense of trust; develops balance, inner strength and focus; strengthens and stretches the legs; softens the spinal muscles; calms the mind.

In this **intimate** upside-down hug, come **closer** together with each deep, **full** breath.

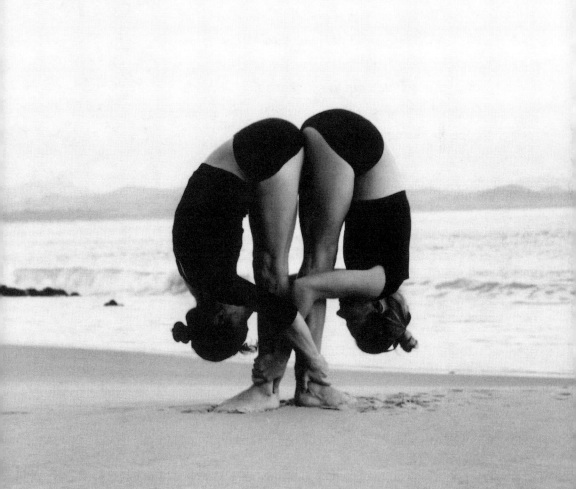

Uttanasana joining

UTTANA–EXTENSION

In the posture: Stand facing your partner about a yard apart. One person bends forward and down, and then the other does the same. The second person to hang forward must slide in from the side, locking their back and head together with their partner's. One at a time, wrap your arms around to reach your partner's ankles. Be very aware of your movements so you don't unbalance each other.

Breathe: Inhale and exhale fully and deeply in unison.

Focus: Stretch out the back of your legs; move in close to each other for a more intense opening.

Hold: 5–10 deep, full breaths. To release, slide out and up one at a time.

Benefits: Develops balance and coordination; stretches the back of the legs; softens the spine; increases blood flow to the brain.

A challenging position where balance and cooperation are the keys for the forward stretch.

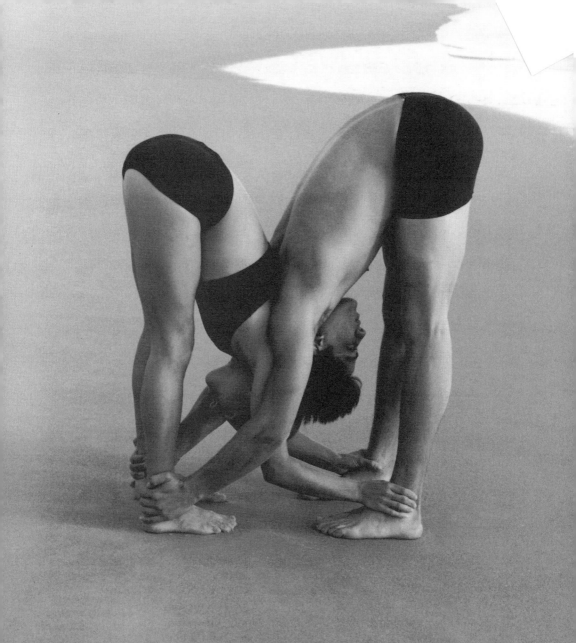

Sitting postures promote calmness of mind and emotions, and have a soothing effect on the systems of the body. There are many ways to support and be with your partner in the sitting postures. Simply breathing together in the postures creates a harmonious practice, increasing sensitivity and awareness.

With the hips and buttocks supported on the ground, we have a stable foundation from which to move. Lengthening and twisting the spine, arms and legs becomes more effortless, and requires less energy than the more dynamic standing postures.

Assist each other to develop length and flexibility in the forward bends, encourage awareness in different parts of the body with simple touch, and apply weight for deeper opening and releasing.

Following are a variety of postures for partner practice. They include postures to develop deep breathing, to open the chest, heart and lungs, to lengthen and tone the limbs, and to tone the nervous system. Others will massage and cleanse the internal organs, stimulate digestion and activate the metabolism. Begin your practice by connecting with each other in the breath.

Sitting well

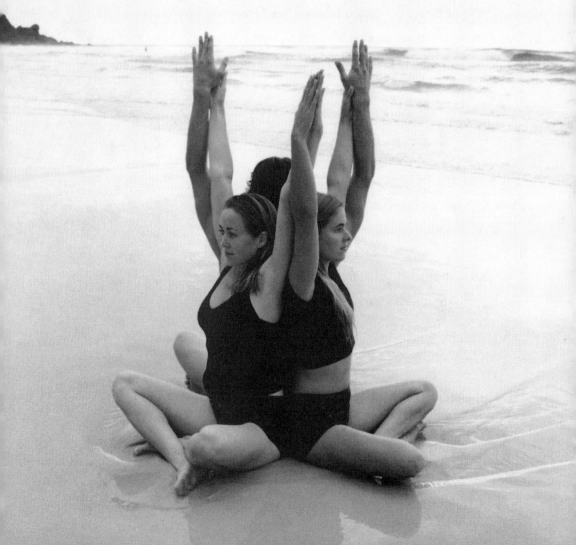

Sukhasana sequence

SUKHA—HAPPY

In the posture: Sit in a comfortable position, back to back with your partner, your arms extended at shoulder height, pressing your palms against your partner's. Breathe together. On the inhalation, slowly raise your arms together, lifting your chest, opening your heart and lungs. On the exhalation, slowly release your arms down. Maintain soft eye gaze straight ahead.

Breathe: Take deep, full, even breaths together.

Focus: Synchronize the movement of your arms with your breathing. Keep your spine extending upwards and your back straight.

Practice: 5–10 cycles to connect with your partner.

Benefits: Develops synchronization of movements with a partner; promotes deep, even breathing; calms the mind and the nervous system.

Synchronize your arm movements with your breath to create a rhythmic flow.

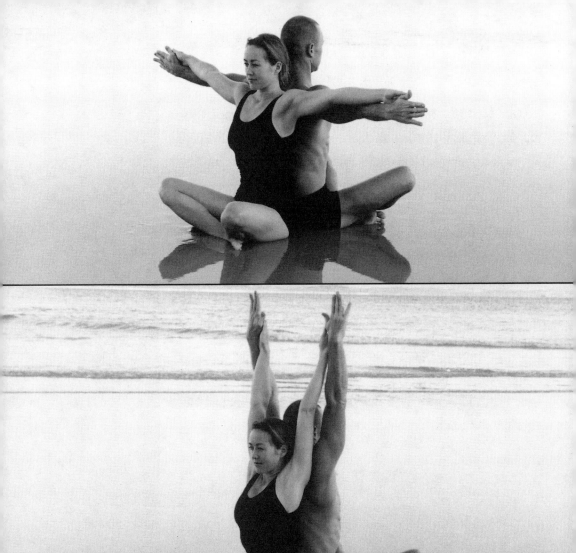

Navasana balance

NAVA—BOAT

In the posture: Sit opposite your partner, legs outstretched. Raise your legs and bring your feet together. Hold each other's hands around the outside of your legs. On the inhalation breath, pull back away from each other and straighten your legs until they are fully extended. If you cannot come up this way, raise one leg at a time, joining your feet at the top. Draw your lower back in, creating a strong, straight back, and activate your abdominal muscles to support you in the pose. Maintain a central point of balance as you pull away from each other.

Breathe: Soft, even, synchronized breathing.

Focus: Concave your lower back; maintain soft eye focus on each other.

Hold: 5–10 deep, full breaths, then release, rest and repeat twice.

Benefits: Tones the spinal nerves; strengthens the abdominal muscles, spine, legs and arms; activates the abdominal organs and stimulates digestion; promotes a sense of balance, coordination and focus.

Floating in calm, mirroring each other's strength, focus and balance.

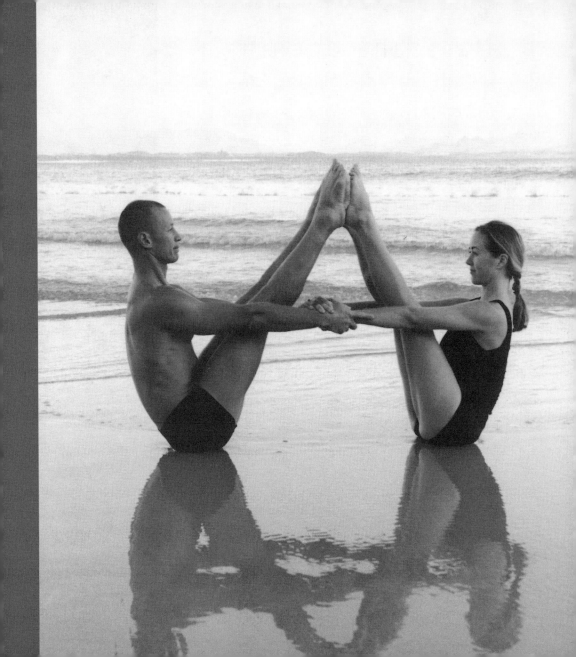

Navasana opening

NAVA–BOAT

In the posture: Sit opposite your partner, your legs outstretched. Raise your feet up to meet each other's, bringing your hands together between your legs. Keeping a firm grip with your hands, pull away from each other, straightening your legs and locking your feet against each other. Draw your lower back in and up, and keep your back straight. Maintain a soft eye gaze with your partner.

Breathe: Inhale and exhale softly and evenly.

Focus: Keep your lower back pulled in, your spine lifting and your legs locked.

Hold: 5–10 deep, full breaths, then release, rest and repeat twice.

Benefits: Strengthens the abdominal muscles and activates the abdominal organs; stimulates digestion; tones the spinal nerves and strengthens the spinal muscles; strengthens the legs and arms; promotes a sense of balance, coordination and focus.

Extending up and outward, create **equilibrium** with grace.

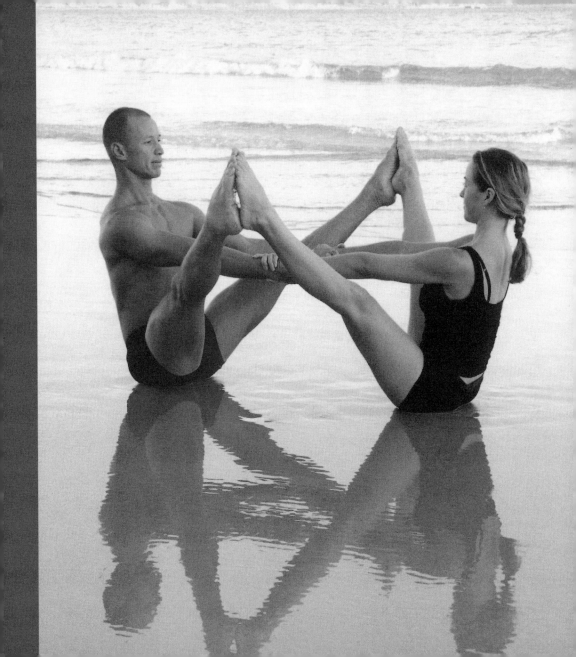

Janu sirsasana adjustment

JANU—KNEE: SIRSA—HEAD

In the posture: One partner sits with their legs outstretched. Bend your right leg, placing the heel of your foot into your groin. Open the sole of the right foot to face upward. Keep the left leg extended outward with the back of the knee pressing into the floor, the left foot flexed and toes drawn back toward the hip. Inhale to lift the front of your body, exhale to soften and release forward and down over your left leg. Hold onto the outside of your foot or wherever you comfortably reach. Rest forehead to knee and gaze toward your toes.

Adjuster: Kneel behind your partner. Place one hand on their right knee to open the hip. Rotate their torso so it lengthens along their outstretched leg.

Breathe: Inhale to lift and lengthen; exhale to soften and release.

Focus: Communicate with your partner about the adjustment.

Hold: 5–10 breaths, then inhale to come up and change sides.

Variation: If you cannot reach your foot, loop a belt around it.

Benefits: Stretches the hamstring muscles and opens the hips; encourages blood flow to the pelvis and reproductive organs; tones the abdominal organs; tones the liver and kidneys; soothes the nervous system; relieves backache.

Encourage your partner to deepen in the releasing with gentle pressure from your hands.

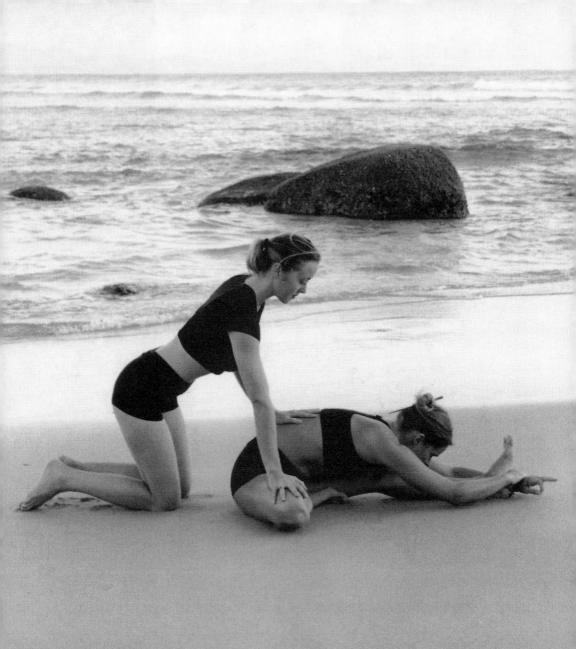

Triang mukhaikapada back stretch

TRI—THREE; ANGA—LIMB; MUKHA—FACE EKA PADA—ONE FOOT

In the posture: One partner sits with their legs outstretched. Bend your right leg back so that the inner part of your foot sits beside your right hip, sole facing upward. Roll your right calf muscle out. Press your left knee to the floor and flex the left foot. Take a deep breath in, lifting the front of your body. As you exhale, lengthen out over your outstretched leg, holding onto the outside of your foot with your hands. Release your forehead to your knee, eye gaze to your foot.

Adjuster: Kneel behind your partner. Place one hand on their right sacrum and hip area, gently working their right buttock down. Place your left hand on their back to encourage extension forward. Rotate their torso so it is lengthening straight along their outstretched leg.

Breathe: Inhale to lift and lengthen forward; exhale to release.

Focus: Keep your hips balanced as you extend forward.

Hold: 5–10 breaths, then inhale to come up and change sides.

Variation: If you cannot reach your foot, loop a belt around it.

Benefits: Stretches the hamstrings; tones the legs' nerves; stretches the spinal muscles; massages the abdominal organs and tones the internal organs; aids in weight loss.

Balance your hips and rejuvenate your spine in this calming forward stretch.

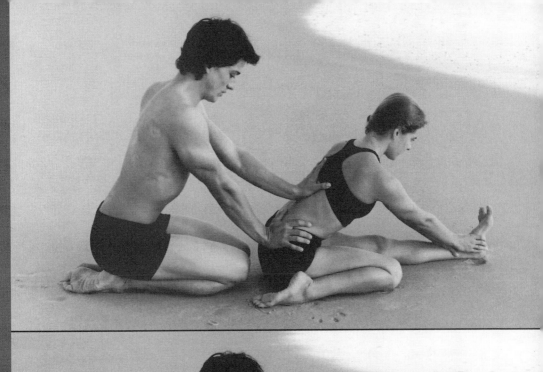

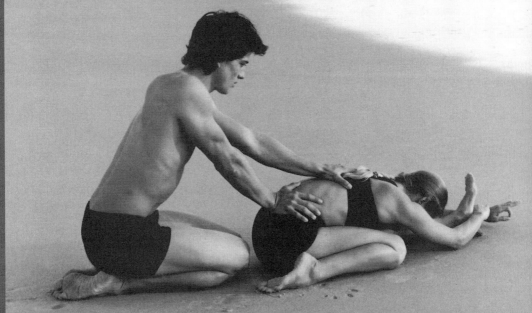

Shoulder release

In the posture: One partner sits in a comfortable position. Inhale to raise your left arm up and place that hand down your back. Next, bring your right arm around your side and join your hands together behind your back. Work the left elbow away from the back of your head. Keep your head upright and keep soft eye gaze forward.

Adjuster: Kneel behind your partner. Place a hand on each elbow and, as your partner is softening with their breath, move them closer together. Communicate about the adjustment, asking if the stretch is strong enough.

Breathe: Focus on breathing fully into the chest.

Focus: Soften into the shoulder opening with the exhalation.

Hold: 5–10 breaths, then release and repeat on the other side. Then swap positions with your partner.

Variation: If your hands do not meet, hold one end of a belt with each hand and focus on drawing the belt in closer together. Your partner can assist you.

Benefits: Releases shoulder tension; lifts and opens the chest and improves breathing.

Release deeply stored, built-up tension in this shoulder opening.

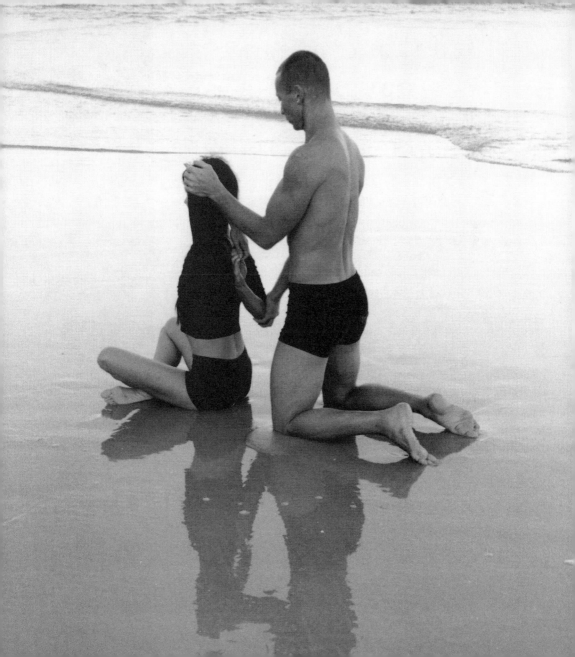

Baddha konasana
opening

BADDHA–BOUND; KONA–ANGLE

In the posture: One partner sits up straight with the soles of their feet together. Interlock your fingers around your toes, and lift out of your lower back. Roll your shoulders down and back, and open your chest. Let the muscles around your hips and pelvis soften and your knees relax to the floor.

Adjuster: Kneel behind your partner. Get in touch with their breathing, inhaling and exhaling as they do. As you exhale together, gently apply pressure to their thighs or knees, assisting them to release their knees to the floor and open their hips. Only go as far as is comfortable for your partner.

Breathe: Inhale and exhale in unison to assist in sensitive adjustment and protect against over adjusting.

Focus: Release and open the hips on the exhalation breath.

Hold: 10 deep, full breaths, then release and swap positions.

Benefits: Tones the kidneys; strengthens the bladder and uterus; opens the hip muscles and relieves pelvic congestion; stimulates blood flow to the reproductive organs and helps to relieve premenstrual tension.

Open up to life, love and creation as you release deeply from the hips and pelvis.

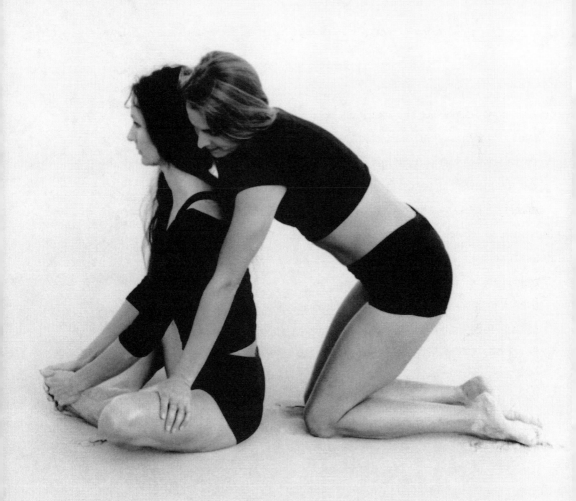

Forward baddha konasana

BADDHA – BOUND; KONA – ANGLE

In the posture: One partner sits up straight with the soles of their feet together. Open your feet out, with only the little-toe sides touching. Interlock your fingers around your toes and lift out of your waist. Let the muscles of your hips soften and your knees relax down toward the floor. As you inhale, lift the front of your body up and extend forward. As you exhale, release your torso forward and down toward the floor, keeping your back extending straight. Rest your forehead down.

Adjuster: Kneel behind your partner and place your hands on their thighs or knees. Begin to breathe with them. As they exhale, apply gentle pressure to their knees to help release their hips.

Breathe: Inhale and exhale together for deep releasing.

Focus: Soften in the hips and release any tension with the exhalation.

Hold: 10–25 deep, full breaths, then release, rest and swap positions.

Variation: Apply pressure to their back for deeper forward extension.

Benefits: Tones the kidneys; strengthens the bladder and uterus; opens the hip muscles and relieves pelvic congestion; stimulates blood flow to the reproductive organs and helps to relieve premenstrual tension; cools the head and calms the mind.

With each breath, feel **healing** oxygenated blood **replenishing** your pelvic and **reproductive** organs.

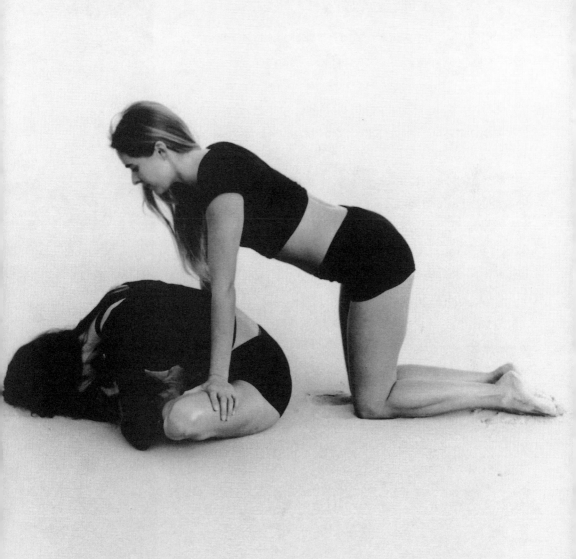

Soft opening

In the posture: One partner sits with the soles of their feet together. Let your knees drop toward the floor and your hips open. As you inhale, lift out of your waist and begin to extend forward from the front of your body. As you exhale, release down, extending your arms forward and gently dropping your head. Soften into the hip opening with each exhalation breath.

Adjuster: Sit back to back with your partner, your legs crossed comfortably. Inhale to raise your arms, tucking your thumbs into the crease of your elbows. When your partner is ready for some weight, lie back over their back and rest your arms and head on their back, tucking your chin in. Be careful not to bear down on them too heavily. Communicate with each other in the adjustment.

Breathe: As you inhale, lift and extend forward; as you exhale, soften and release deeper into the hips.

Focus: Concentrate on releasing in the hips and lengthening through your back.

Hold: For as long as is comfortable or 10–20 deep, full breaths. To come up, the adjuster releases first. Then swap positions with your partner.

Benefits: Both postures open the hips and encourage circulation to the pelvic and reproductive organs. The adjuster receives an opening in the chest, heart and lungs.

Allow your **partner's** weight to help you enter melting **calm**.

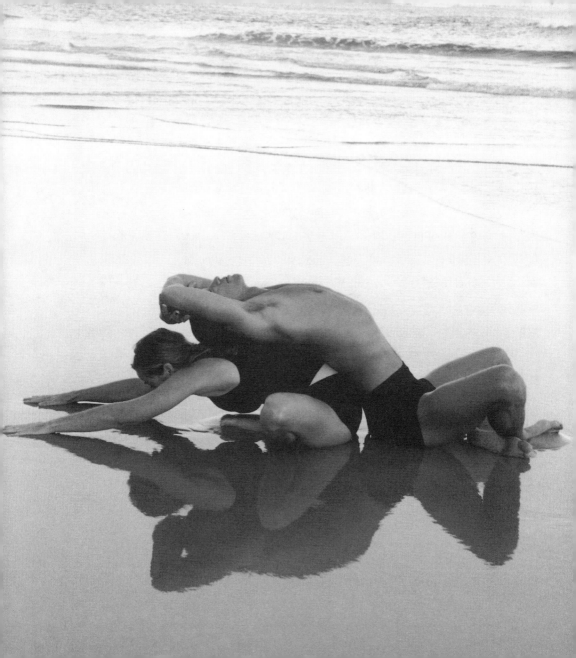

Padmasana yoking

PADMA—LOTUS

In the posture: Sit facing your partner in full lotus position (your right foot sits on top of your left thigh and your left foot on top of your right thigh, crossing over the right leg). Draw your knees in close together and your feet in close to your groin, flexing your feet. Put your arms behind you on the floor, lean back into them and raise your knees off the floor. Wriggle in close to your partner so that your buttocks and legs press together. One at a time, wrap your arms around your partner's shoulders and draw into each other to form an egg shape with your two bodies. Gaze softly at your partner.

Breathe: Take slow, even breaths though your nose.

Focus: Lift out of your lower back, keeping your knees close together.

Hold: 5–10 breaths, or as long as is comfortable, then release and cross the legs the opposite way to repeat, or move straight into *Flowering Padmasana*, on the next page.

Benefits: Stretches the knee joints; opens the hips; stimulates blood flow to the pelvic region.

Note: Only attempt this posture if you're able to sit in *Padmasana* comfortably.

Two **halves** create a **whole** in this beautifully bound **embrace.**

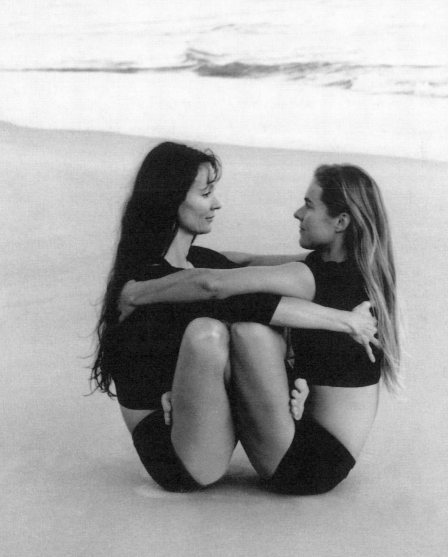

Flowering padmasana

PADMA—LOTUS

In the posture: Position into *Padmasana Yoking*, on the previous page, this time with the arms extended and holding each other's upper arms. Take a deep inhalation together, and on the exhalation drop your head back, pulling away from each other. You may need to release your arms a little. Open your chest, heart and lungs and stretch your throat as you gaze back to your third eye (the point between your eyebrows).

Breathe: Take deep, full breaths.

Focus: Lift out of your lower back, opening and lifting your chest.

Hold: 5–10 breaths, or as long as is comfortable, then exhale to release. Cross your legs the other way and repeat.

Benefits: Stretches the knee joints; opens the hips; stimulates blood flow to the pelvic region; opens the chest and stretches the throat.

Opening out to life, a blooming flower sprouting from a stable base.

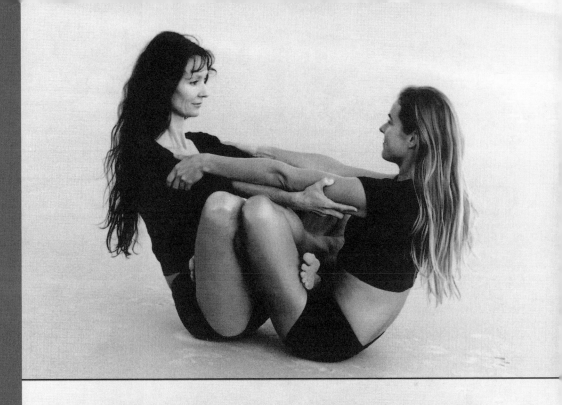
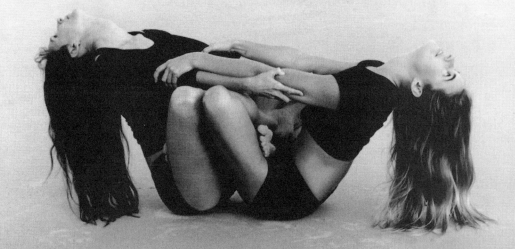

United konasana

KONA—ANGLE

In the posture: Sit on the floor facing each other with your legs spread wide. The adjustee activates their legs and presses the backs of their knees to the floor. Focus on tilting the pelvis forward and lengthening the torso down.

Adjuster: Bend your knees and position your feet on your partner's inner legs, between their ankles and knees. Lean forward and hold onto your partner's elbows. As your partner releases forward, work with the breath and pull their arms. Encourage them to lengthen and apply some pressure to their legs, sliding them open for a deeper release in the groin and inner leg muscles.

Breathe: Inhale and exhale deeply and fully in unison with each other.

Focus: Be sensitive in the adjustment to avoid overstretching.

Hold: 5–10 deep full breaths, softening into the opening with each exhalation, then release and change positions.

Variation: Rest your buttocks on the edge of a folded blanket to assist in the forward pelvic tilt. If you cannot lean forward, sit upright and focus on the opening in your leg and groin muscles.

Benefits: Releases the groin and inner leg muscles; relieves pelvic congestion; stimulates circulation to the pelvic and reproductive organs and helps to regulate the menstrual cycle.

Softening open with deep full breaths, feel yourself yielding and letting go.

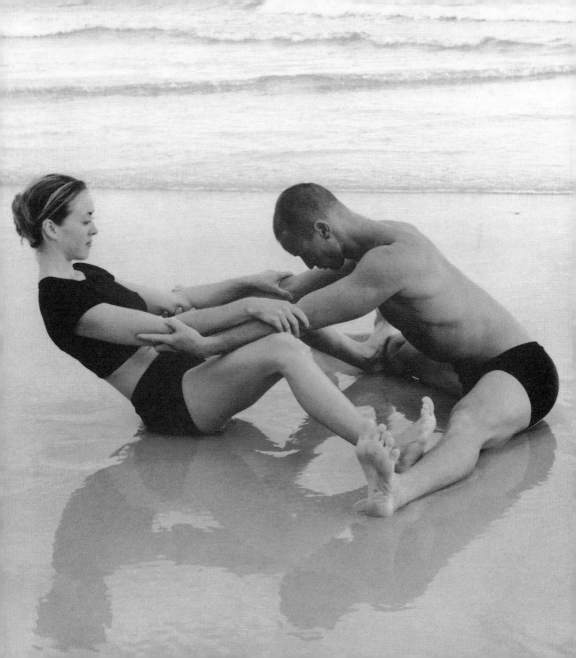

Konasana
forward adjustment

KONA–ANGLE

In the posture: One partner sits with legs wide apart and back straight. Flex your feet and push out through the balls and heels, extending the backs of your legs. Press the backs of your knees to the ground. On an inhalation, lift out of your waist and slowly come forward, lifting your abdomen and chest as you extend. As you exhale, release down, relaxing your head, neck and facial muscles. Extend your arms out in front of you, palms to the floor. Keep the backs of your legs pressing into the ground and kneecaps in line with your feet.

Adjuster: Place your hands on their lower back to release them further forward with each exhalation breath.

Breathe: Extend forward with the inhalation, soften fully with the exhalation.

Focus: Softening in the inner leg and groin muscles.

Hold: 10 deep, full breaths, then release and swap positions.

Variation: Rest your buttocks on the edge of a folded blanket to assist in the forward pelvic tilt.

Benefits: Opens the hips and releases tension and tight muscles in the groin and inner leg; encourages blood flow to the pelvic and reproductive organs and helps regulate the menstrual cycle.

Melting forward and down, surrender and soften into a space of endless opening and freedom.

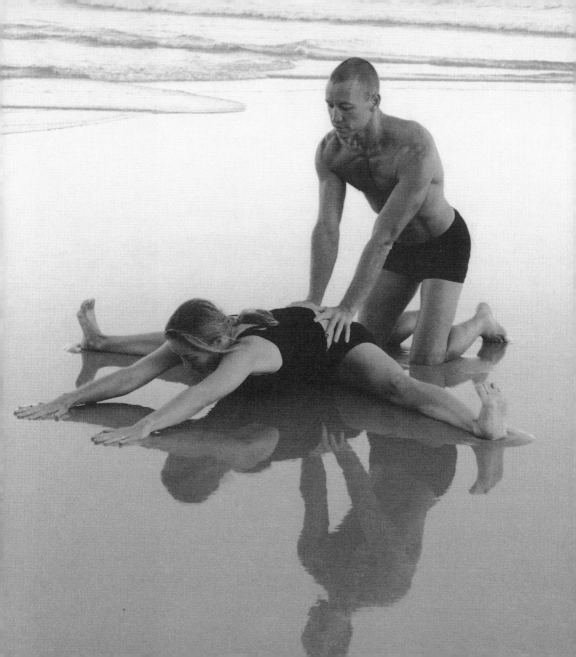

Side-cupped konasana

KONA—ANGLE

In the posture: Sit in a wide-legged position, cupped with your partner so your legs, hips and back are merging. Activate your legs and work the backs of your knees to the floor. Flex your feet, turning your toes back toward your head. Breathing in unison, inhale to lift out of your waist and turn to face your right leg. Together with your partner, extend forward and over your right leg, and hold your own and your partner's foot. The person at the back lies over the front person.

Breathe: Inhale and exhale together. As you inhale, lift and extend forward from the front of your body. As you exhale, release forward and down.

Focus: Keep your legs activated and toes turning back toward your hips. Soften in the inner leg and groin muscles with the out breath.

Hold: 5–10 deep, full breaths, then release and move to the left leg.

Benefits: Stretches the hamstrings; opens and softens the inner leg muscles; stimulates flow of blood to the pelvic and reproductive organs; extends and softens the spinal muscles.

Softening forwards, lengthen beyond limitations with deep, full breathing.

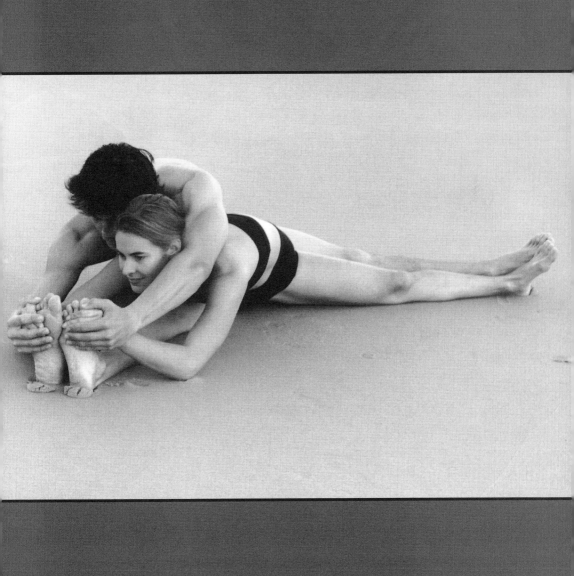

Malasana link

MALA - GARLAND

In the posture: Squat back to back with your partner. Bring your own feet together and knees apart. Lean forward between your knees, bringing your arms around the outside of your lower legs to hold your partner's hands. Release your torso through your legs as you soften and rest forward. Use the grip of your partner's hands to pull away and lengthen the torso forward more.

Breathe: Inhale to lift and expand the chest, exhale to soften and release the torso through the legs.

Focus: Soften the hips and work the heels to the ground.

Hold: 5–10 breaths.

Benefits: Stretches the ankles and legs; opens the hips; stimulates blood flow to the pelvic and reproductive organs; releases tension in the lower back.

Linked back to back, two bodies entwine for mutual lengthening and releasing.

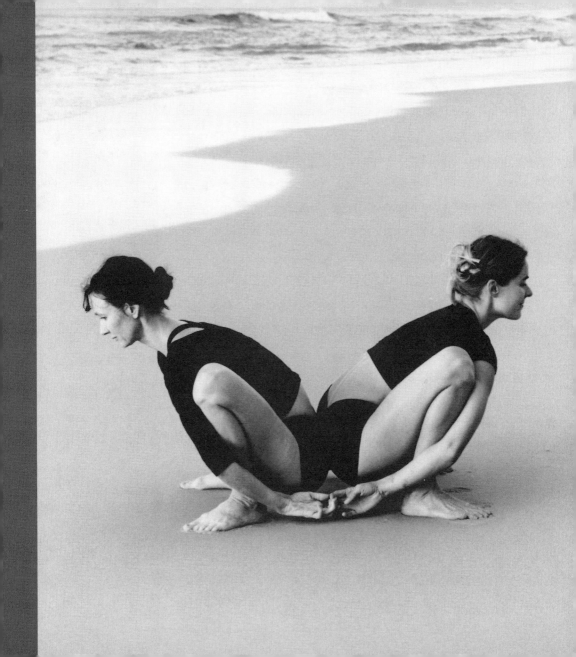

Kurmasana softening

KURMA—TORTOISE

In the posture: One partner begins, sitting with the soles of their feet together. Slide your feet forward and place your hands under your knees. Hang your torso down and bring your hands under your legs to meet your feet. Release down, relaxing your head, shoulders and spine. As you exhale, soften in the groin, hip and inner leg muscles.

Adjuster: Kneel behind your partner, placing your hands along their back. Applying weight, encourage their shoulders to move downward and their head, neck and back to soften and release.

Breathe: Inhale and exhale deeply and fully through the nose, focusing on letting go of tension with the exhalation.

Focus: Let go and soften in the hip and groin muscles.

Hold: 10 deep, full breaths, then release and change positions.

Benefits: Strengthens the back; releases the inner leg, hip and groin muscles; stimulates blood flow to the pelvic and reproductive organs and relieves pelvic congestion; soothes the nerves in the legs.

Hang forward, disappearing inward where the mind quiets and the body rests.

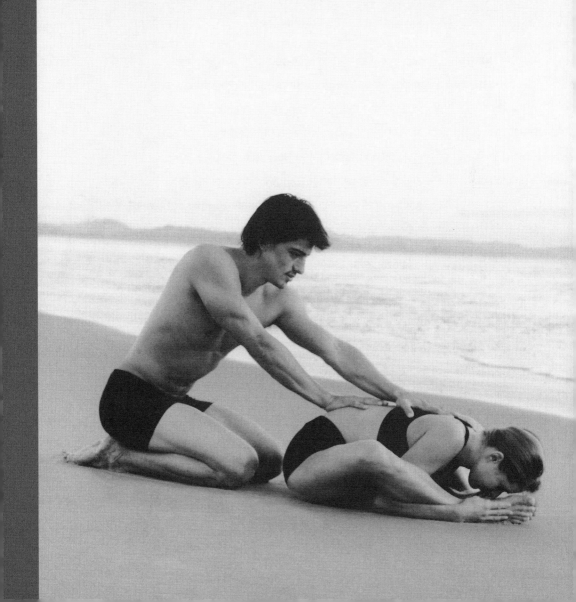

Pascimottanasana I & II

PASCIMA–BACK: UTTANA–EXTENSION

In the posture: Sit opposite your partner with your legs outstretched and your feet pressing against theirs. Move the flesh of your buttocks away so you're on your sitting bones, pelvis tilting forward. Activate and contract the muscles of the front of your leg, drawing your kneecaps and thighs up, pressing the backs of your knees to the floor. Flex your feet, pressing the soles into your partner's and drawing the toes back toward the hips. From this foundation, inhale to lift out of the waist, lifting your abdomen and chest and extending forward over your legs. Place your hands onto your feet and hold your partner's hands there. Keep your back straight and your chest lifted as you focus on lengthening your back and legs. If you have the flexibility, move into *Pascimottanasana II* by inhaling to lift and extend, and exhaling to soften and release down. Slide your arms along your partner's and use the grip to pull yourself forward.

Breathe: Inhale to lift the whole front of the body, exhale to soften forward and down.

Focus: Keep your back lengthening, not rounding, as you come forward.

Hold: 10–20 breaths, or for as long as is comfortable.

Benefits: Separates the spinal vertebrae; increases circulation throughout the body; promotes a healthy, supple back; soothes the nervous system; stretches the legs; stimulates digestion, calms the mind.

Assist each other to extend forward and release down into a quiet internal space.

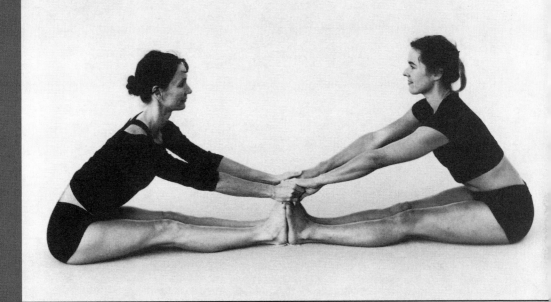

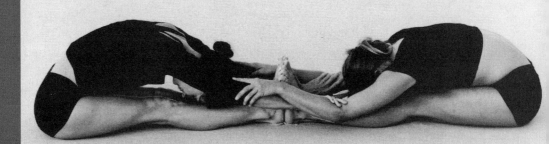

Pascimottanasana adjustment

PASCIMA—BACK; UTTANA—EXTENSION

In the posture: Sit with your legs outstretched. Move the flesh of your buttocks away so you're on your sitting bones. Activate and contract the muscles of the front of your leg and press the backs of your knees to the floor. Flex your feet, pressing the balls and heels away. Inhale to lift out of the waist, extending forward. Place your hands on the outside of your feet and exhale to release down, resting your forehead to your legs. Eye gaze towards your feet.

Adjuster: Kneel behind your partner, encourage the stretch by applying gentle pressure to their lower back, moving their spine up as they lengthen.

Breathe: In unison, inhale to lift and extend, exhale to release.

Focus: Keep your knees pressed to the floor, feet and legs activated, toes working back towards your head.

Hold: 5–10 deep, full breaths, then release and swap positions.

Variation: If you cannot rest forward, hold a belt looped around your feet and sit upright with the lower back concaving. Lengthen your spine, drawing your lower back in and relaxing your shoulders down.

Benefits: Softens the spine and spinal muscles; extends and stretches the backs of the legs; strengthens the fronts of the legs; calms the nervous system; encourages an inward focus and calms the mind.

The mind succumbs to the calm of turning inward, away from activity.

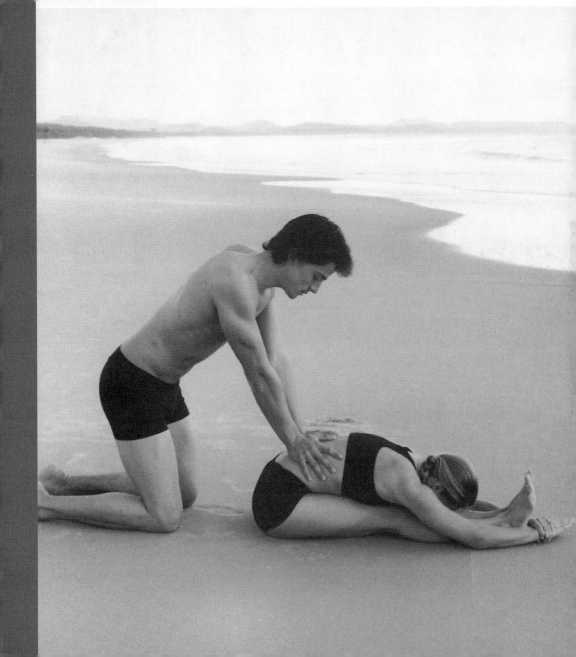

Pascimottanasana deep adjustment

PASCIMA–BACK; UTTANA–EXTENSION

In the posture: One partner begins, sitting with their legs outstretched. Move the flesh of your buttocks away so you're on your sitting bones. Activate and contract the muscles of the front of your legs, draw your kneecaps and thighs up, press the backs of your knees to the floor and flex your feet. Inhale to lift out of the waist, lifting your abdomen and chest and extending forward. Place your hands around the outside of your feet and exhale to release, resting your forehead to your legs. Eyes gaze towards your feet.

Adjuster: When your partner is fully in the pose, lie the front of your torso over their back, holding their feet and moving your body weight forward and upwards, helping them to lengthen their torso forward.

Breathe: Inhale to lift and extend, exhale to soften and release.

Focus: Keep your knees pressed to the floor, feet and legs activated, toes working back towards your head.

Hold: 5–10 deep, full breaths, then release and swap positions.

Benefits: Softens the spine and spinal muscles; extends and stretches the backs of the legs; strengthens the fronts of the legs; calms the nervous system.

With the weight of your **partner** on your back, sink **deep** into the release and **opening**.

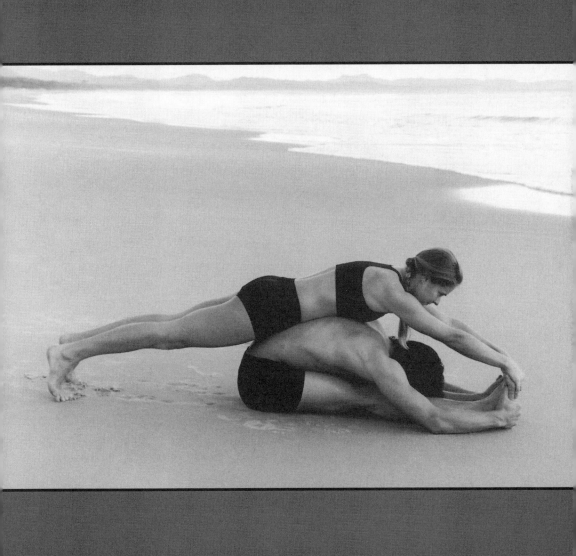

Pascimottanasana back to back adjustment

PASCIMA—BACK; UTTANA—EXTENSION

In the posture: One partner sits with legs outstretched and activated. Press the backs of the knees to the ground and flex the toes back towards your hips. Draw the muscles of the front of the legs upwards. Inhale to lift the front of your body up, exhale to lengthen forward and lie down over your outstretched legs. Rest your forehead down and focus on the breath to soften and release in the pose.

Adjuster: Sit back to back with your partner, your legs crossed comfortably. When your partner is ready for adjustment, lie back over their back, positioning yourself so you are assisting your partner to lengthen through the spine. Rest your back, head and shoulders on their back. Be careful not to bear down on your partner with too much weight. Communicate with each other to make sure the adjustment is working.

Breathe: Inhale to lift and extend, exhale to soften and release.

Focus: Keep your legs locked and lengthening forward. Relax.

Hold: 5–10 deep, full breaths, then release and swap positions.

Benefits: Softens the spinal muscles and stretches the spine; stretches the hamstrings; strengthens the fronts of the legs; massages the abdominal organs and stimulates digestion.

One person lies forward, journeying inward, while the other relaxes backwards and opens outward.

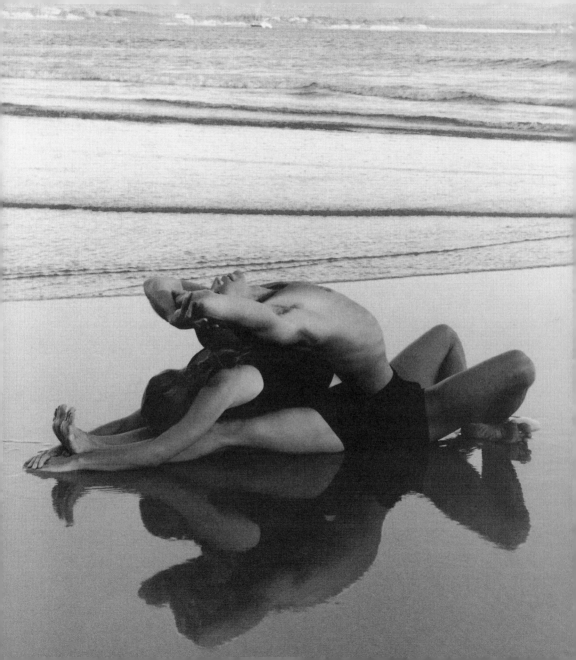

Simhasana

SIMHA—LION

In the posture: Kneel facing each other, your knees wide apart and your buttocks on your heels. Slide your heels out to the sides so that your buttocks release onto the floor between your heels. Place your hands between your knees, fingers facing inward towards your body and palms down. Lean forward into your wrists and drop your head back. Open your mouth wide, poking your tongue out as far as possible. Direct your eye gaze to your third eye (the point between your eyebrows). Inhale deeply through your nose, and on the exhale produce an "Ah" sound from deep in your throat. Inhale through your nose again, and exhale with a roaring sound from the mouth (hence the name, lion's pose).

Breathe: Inhale fully, then exhale with a roar.

Focus: Produce a strong "Ah" sound from the throat.

Practice: 5–10 cycles, or for as long as is comfortable.

Benefits: Clears and cleanses the throat and passages of the ears, nose and mouth; promotes a clear voice; develops good speech and confidence.

Through the release of roaring "Ahs," the sweetness of our voice is uncovered.

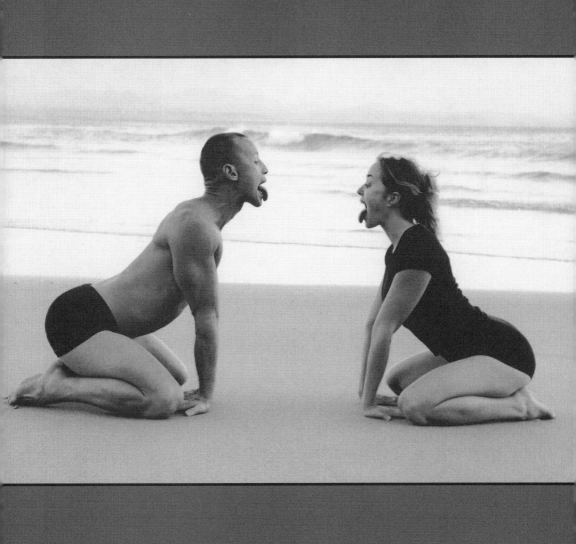

Supta padangusthasana leg stretch

SUPTA—SUPINE; PADANGUSTHA—BIG TOE

In the posture: One partner lies on their back, legs outstretched. Tuck your chin in, and as you inhale, raise your right leg, holding your big toe with the first two fingers of your right hand. As you breathe, soften your right leg forward and down towards your torso. Place your left hand on your left hip to keep it down.

Adjuster: From kneeling, place your right hand on their left leg to keep it down, and your left hand on their right ankle. As they exhale, apply gentle pressure to their right leg, assisting them to release the leg forward and down over their head.

Breathe: Inhale and exhale in unison to increase the releasing.

Focus: Keep the left hip down and the chin tucked in.

Hold: Release in the assisted opening for 5—10 deep breaths, then repeat on the left side. Swap positions with your partner or move straight into *Supta Padangusthasana Side Stretch*.

Variations: Bend your left leg up, placing the foot toward your left buttock for extra support. If you cannot reach your toes, hold a belt looped around your foot.

Benefits: Stretches the hamstrings; releases the hip and lower back muscles; increases strength in the muscles of the fronts of the legs.

Relax your mind and body as tightness melts away with each deep, full breath.

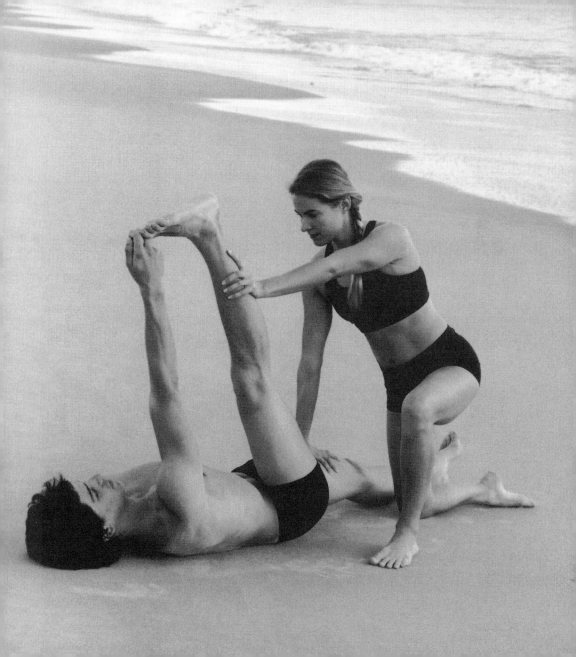

Supta padangusthasana side stretch

SUPTA—SUPINE; PADANGUSTHA—BIG TOE

In the posture: One partner positions into *Supta Padangusthasana Leg Stretch*, on the previous page. From this position, inhale. As you exhale, release your right leg out to the right, resting the foot down. Turn your right heel out to contact the floor first. Keep the muscles of the front of the leg activated, the ball and heel of your foot pushing away from you, and your toes working back towards your head. Stretch out through the back of your leg and contract the front leg muscles. Keep your left hip down to the floor with your left hand.

Adjuster: Assist your partner in releasing by moving their leg down towards the floor and up towards their head. Work with the breath, applying gentle pressure as they exhale. Keep their left hip down to the floor.

Breathe: Synchronize your breathing for deep, sensitive releasing.

Focus: Soften the inner leg muscles with the exhalation.

Hold: 5–10 deep, full breaths. Inhale to release the right leg back to the center. Exhale to release it to the floor and change legs. Then swap positions with your partner.

Benefits: Stretches open the inner leg muscles and softens the hip and groin muscles; stimulates blood flow to the pelvic organs.

With each **deep** breath, **surrender** to a soft space of freedom and **eternal** opening.

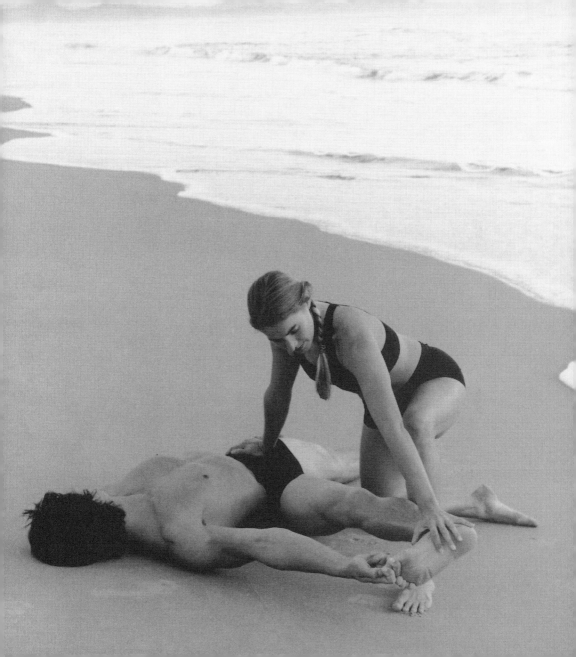

Leg stretch adjustment

In the posture: One partner lies on their back, arms by their sides, palms facing down. When you are ready, inhale to raise your legs off the floor and over your head. Keep your lower back and tail bone in contact with the floor, and draw your abdomen back to your spine. Breathe into the stretch, letting go of tension in the backs of the legs.

Adjuster: Sit on the floor at the top of your partner's head. When your partner has raised their legs to their maximum extension, hold their ankles and, communicating with your partner, slowly begin to draw their feet closer towards the floor above their head. Only take them as far as is comfortable.

Breathe: Take deep, full breaths, releasing and softening into the stretch with the exhalation.

Focus: Keep your lower back to the floor.

Hold: Stay releasing in the pose for 5–10 deep, full breaths. Exhale to release the legs down and swap positions with your partner.

Benefits: A deep opening into the back of the legs, hamstrings and buttock muscles.

Resting back, be in a position to release the legs and let go completely.

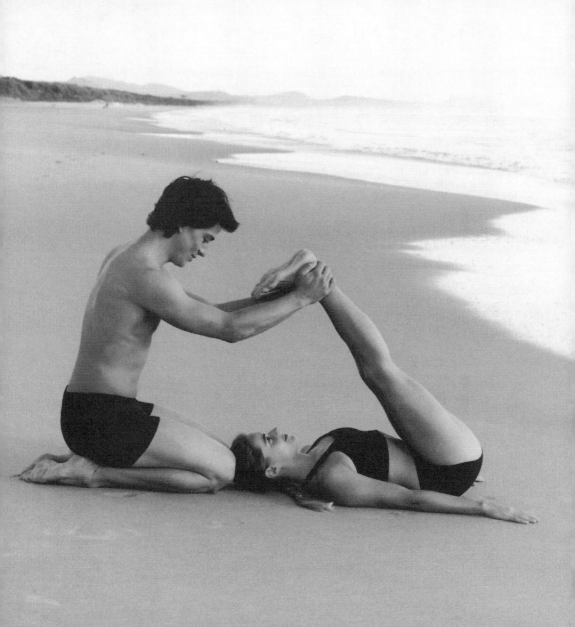

Supported leg lifts

In the posture: One partner lies on their back, arms by their sides, palms facing down and their head resting on their partner's knees. On the inhalation breath, raise your legs to a 90° angle, and with the exhalation breath, release them to the ground. Keep your legs locked and your feet together. Move slowly with the breath and keep your lower back pressing into the floor. Feel your abdominal muscles working. Keep your head and neck relaxed and your arms pressing into the floor.

Adjuster: Sit on the ground, your buttocks to your heels and with your partner's head resting on your knees. Place your hands on their shoulders, and as they bring their legs up and down, keep their shoulders down.

Breathe: Take slow and even breaths. Inhale to raise your legs up, exhale to release them down.

Focus: Use your abdominal muscles to lift. Keep your lower back to the floor as the legs raise, and facial and neck muscles relaxed.

Practice: 3 sets of 10 lifts, or as many as are comfortable. Rest before changing places with your partner.

Variation: Keep your legs bent if you need to or if your lower back is straining.

Benefits: Tones the abdominal muscles and massages the internal organs; tones the muscles and nerves of the legs and hips.

Inspire each other to move from the core with strength and focus.

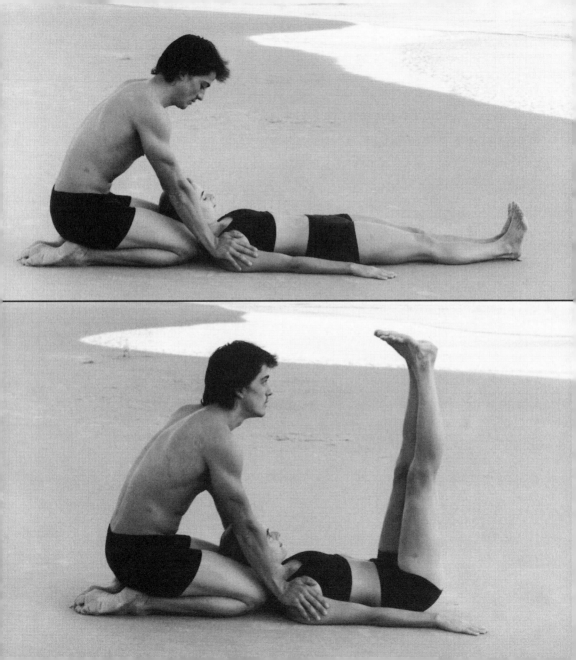

Combined leg lifts

In the posture: Lie down on your backs, head to head but about an arm's length apart. Extend your arms above your head and hold your partner's upper arms. Press your lower back to the floor and draw your abdomen back to your spine. Working together, inhale to raise your legs to a 90° angle, exhale to release them to the floor. As you move, keep your legs locked and feet together. Keep your movements and breathing synchronized with each other. Make the lifts slow and controlled, and focus on working your abdominal muscles.

Breathe: Inhale and exhale in unison with each other.

Focus: Use your abdominal muscles to lift your legs. Keep your head, neck and facial muscles soft.

Practice: 3 sets of 10 cycles, or for as long as is comfortable.

Variation: Keep your knees bent if needed or if your lower back is straining. If you have the strength, keep your feet off the floor throughout the cycles.

Benefits: Strengthens the muscles of the abdomen and massages the abdominal organs; strengthens the legs; develops a harmonious connection with your partner.

A doubles lift combining two energies to build strength and dynamism.

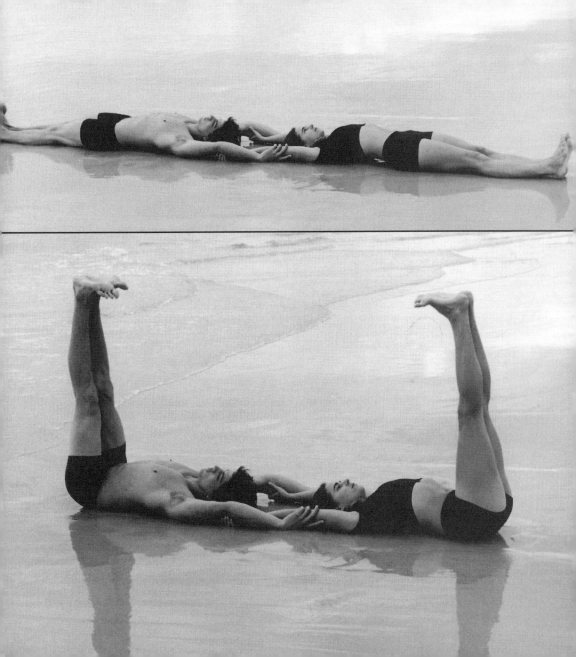

The rejuvenating after-effect of a twist is immediate. Deeply cleansing and therapeutic, twisting postures massage the internal organs, releasing stores of wastes from the body and giving life to its sluggish systems. Enhancing energy levels and vitality, twists are good to practice in the morning when you need to wake up or in the afternoon for an instant pick-me-up.

Because they rotate the spine, twists soften tight muscles. They help remove aches and pains from the back, release neck and shoulder tension and give freedom of movement to tired and tight bodies. As you unlock your body, wastes as well as stored emotions are released. Become aware of the awakened emotions coming to the surface and breathe deeply to release them with the out breath.

With a partner to assist you in the twisting action, your body can go that little bit further, increasing the cleansing effects. Whether together in a pose or adjusting each other, always twist with the breath. Inhale to lift out of the waist and exhale to turn further in the twist. Deep, full breaths will aid in deep twisting and releasing. Communicate with your partner; if the adjustment feels too strong or not strong enough, let your partner know.

With practice, the spinal muscles will soften and flexibility will increase. Only twist as far as is comfortable. Avoid these postures if you suffer from back problems. Do not attempt twisting postures when pregnant.

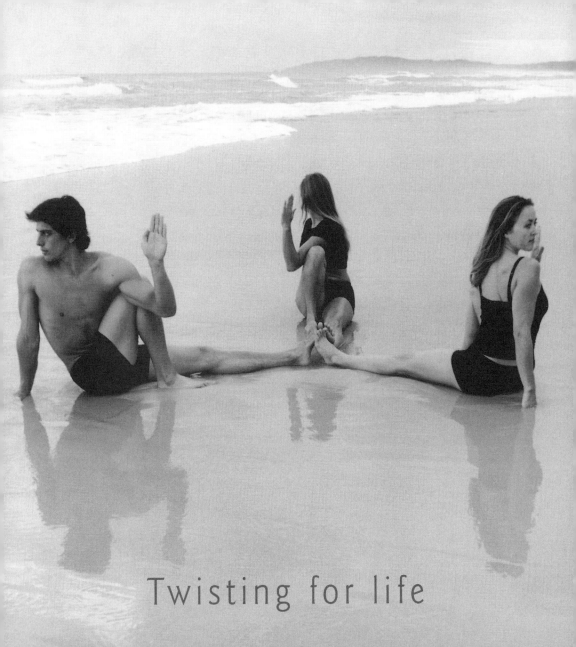

Twisting for life

Sukhasana entwined

SUKHA–HAPPY

In the posture: Sit in a cross-legged position back to back with your partner so that your backs and shoulders are touching. Inhale and lift out of your waist. Exhale and place your left hand on your right knee and stretch your right hand around your back to hold your partner's left knee. Inhale to lift, and thinning your waist, exhale to turn to look over your right shoulder. Your partner will be doing the same twist, so you'll both be turning to look in opposite directions.

Breathe: Inhale and exhale together, twisting deeper with each breath.

Focus: Inhale to lift, exhale to twist.

Hold: 5–10 deep, full breaths, then release and change directions.

Benefits: Massages the abdominal and other internal organs, aiding in digestion and weight loss; stretches the spinal muscles, separates the vertebrae; tones the spinal cord and the nervous system; stimulates blood flow to the pelvis and hips.

Spiraling from the base upwards, rotate around each other, creating an intricate twist.

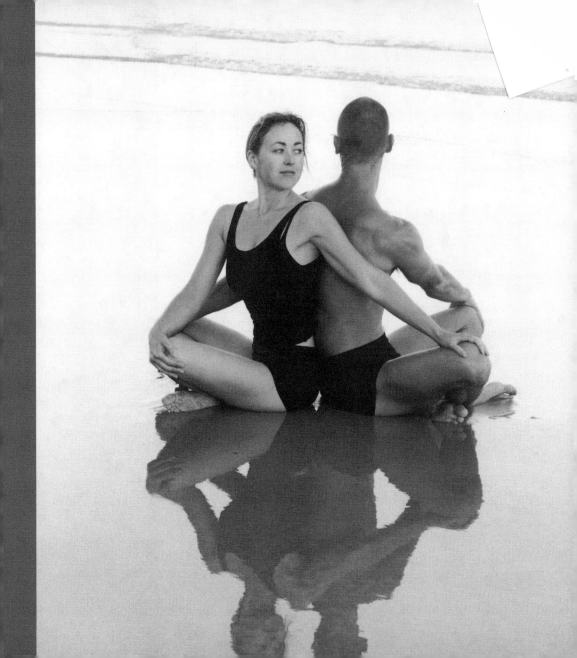

Spinal roll adjustment

In the posture: One partner lies on their back, heels into their buttocks, arms out to their sides at shoulder height, palms facing down. Inhale deeply and on the exhale release your knees to the right, keeping your legs together. Draw your knees close up to your arm and rest your legs on the floor. Turn your head to look over your left shoulder to complete the twist. Keep your shoulders pressing into the floor and breathe deeply into the spinal release.

Adjuster: Kneel beside your partner, placing your left hand on their left hip and your right hand on their left shoulder to keep it to the floor. As they exhale, gently move their left hip further over to the right side while communicating with your partner. Begin gently and ask if they'd like more adjustment. Work with their breath.

Breathe: Take deep, full breaths, releasing deeper with the exhalation.

Focus: Soften the spine and release any tension.

Hold: 10 deep, full breaths, then release your legs back to the center and exhale to drop them over to the left side, your head turning to face the right.

Benefits: Stretches the back muscles and releases tension and tightness; separates the spinal vertebrae and stimulates healthy blood flow; tones the spinal cord; massages deep into the abdominal organs, stimulating metabolism and digestion.

Let go of any tension, release and discover the spine's natural openness and flexibility.

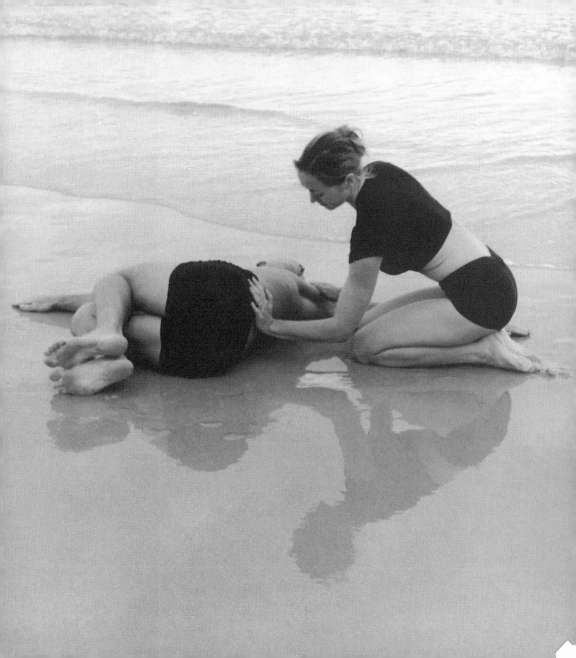

Jathara parivartasana assist

JATHARA—ABDOMEN; PARIVARTANA—TURNING

In the posture: One partner lies on their back, arms out to their sides at shoulder height, palms facing upwards. Have your head centered and face upwards, your chin tucked in. On exhalation, raise your straight legs to a 90° angle. Lift your hips over to the left slightly and, keeping your left shoulder pressing into the floor, slowly release your legs down to your right side so the feet hover above the right hand. Stay in this position for a few breaths, then inhale to release your legs to the center and rest for a few breaths. Repeat on the left-hand side.

Adjuster: Kneel above your partner's head, place your hands on their shoulders and keep them pressed down into the floor.

Breathe: Inhale to lift your legs to the center, exhale to release them to the side.

Focus: Keep your shoulders down and keep your feet off the floor. Keep your torso in line with your hips when your legs are to the side.

Practice: 5–10 cycles, depending on your strength.

Variations: If you cannot hover your feet, rest them on the floor near your outstretched arm. Or keep the bent, knees together.

Benefits: Massages and strengthens the abdominal organs and muscles, stimulating digestion and relieving intestinal disorders.

Wind the abdomen into a deep internal twist, releasing tension and regaining vitality.

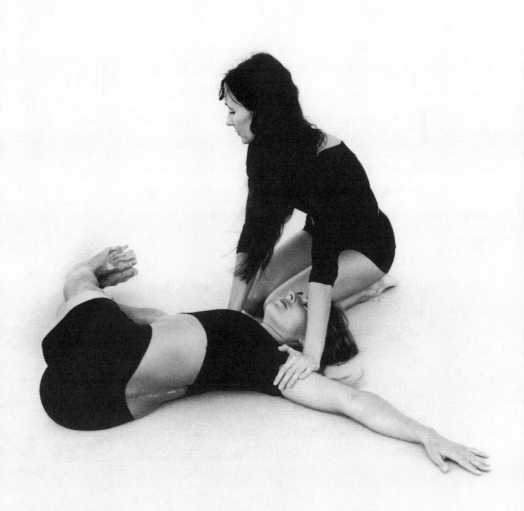

Ardha badhha inside twist

ARDHA—HALF; BADDHA—BOUND

In the posture: Sit side by side with your partner, legs outstretched. Bend your outside leg into half-lotus position, bringing your foot to rest on top of the thigh of your inside leg. Have your inside extended leg touching your partner's. Inhale to lift out of your waist, raising both arms and turning to face your partner. Exhale to extend your outside arm out and hold the outside edge of your partner's foot. Raise your inside arm, pressing the palm of your hand into your partner's to create an upward-pointing arrow. Gaze up at your hands and work in the twist with the breath.

Breathe: Inhale to lift, exhale to turn and lift.

Focus: Keep the knee of your extended leg pressing into the floor and your toes flexing back towards your hips. Release the bent knee to the floor to open your hip.

Hold: 5–10 deep, full breaths, then release and repeat on the other leg.

Variation: If it strains your knee to have it in the half-lotus position, rest that foot on the floor beside your thigh instead of on top of it.

Benefits: Stretches the spinal muscles; releases a tight back and tension; stimulates the spinal cord and improves suppleness in the back; opens the hips, chest, heart and lungs.

Aim for new heights in this intricate opening for the spine, legs, chest and shoulders.

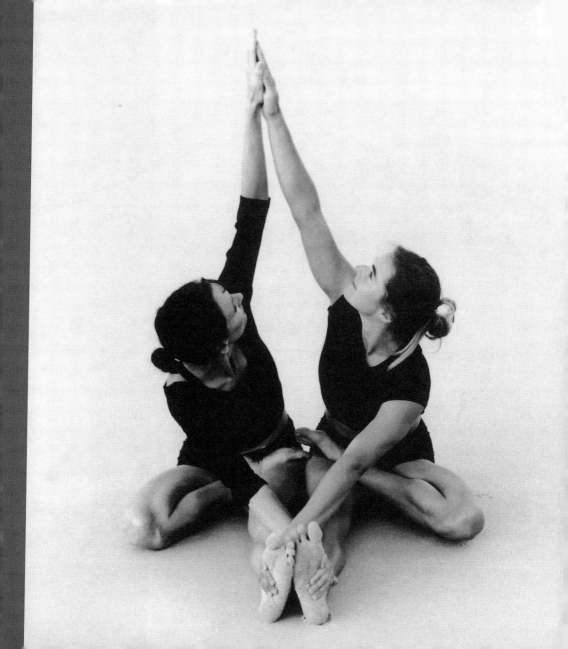

Maricyasana rotation

MARICI—AN INDIAN SAGE

In the posture: One partner sits on the floor, legs outstretched. Bend your right leg and place the foot close to your groin so that your right thigh is against your abdomen. Inhale and turn to place your right hand on the floor behind your right hip. Lock your left arm in front of your right knee, pressing your arm into your knee. Inhale and lift out of your hips, thinning your waist. Exhale and turn to look over your right shoulder, tucking in your chin. Keep your left leg straight, and the back of the knee pressing into the floor.

Adjuster: Sit behind your partner and place your right hand on their right shoulder and your left hand on their waist above their left hip. As they inhale to lift, lift their torso upwards; as they exhale to twist, assist the rotation by turning their right shoulder out and rotating their left waist around toward the front.

Breathe: Inhale deeply then release fully on the exhalation.

Focus: Release tension and tightness in the spine.

Hold: 5–10 deep, full breaths, then release and twist to the other side. Then swap positions with your partner.

Benefits: Stretches and tones the spinal cord; massages and cleanses the internal organs; relieves a sore back and releases tension in the spine; stimulates metabolism and refreshes the brain.

A highly effective twist to cleanse sluggish systems and give a refreshing pick-me-up.

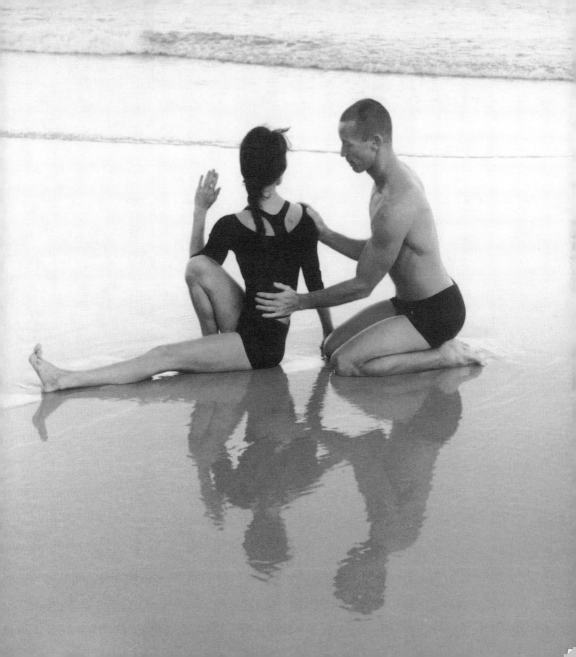

Maricyasana deep release

MARICI—AN INDIAN SAGE

In the posture: Sit facing your partner, legs side by side and outstretched. Bend your right leg and place the foot close to your groin so that your right thigh is against your abdomen. The foot of your extended leg rests to the side of your partner's right hip. Inhale to lift out of your waist, exhale to turn to look over your right shoulder. Lock your left arm in front of your right knee and extend it out to hold your partner's right hand. Bring your right hand around your back and hold your partner's extended left hand. Pull your partner's hands to increase each other's stretch and twist in the pose.

Breathe: Inhale to lift, exhale to twist.

Focus: Thin your waist as you inhale, release any tension in the spine as you exhale.

Hold: 10 breaths, or for as long as is comfortable, then release and repeat on the other side.

Variation: If you cannot reach each other's hands, sit closer together or use a belt to join the gap.

Benefits: Stretches and tones the spinal cord; massages and cleanses the internal organs; relieves a sore back and releases tension in the spine; stimulates the metabolism and refreshes the brain.

Join hands and rotate together for deep releasing, cleansing and rejuvenating.

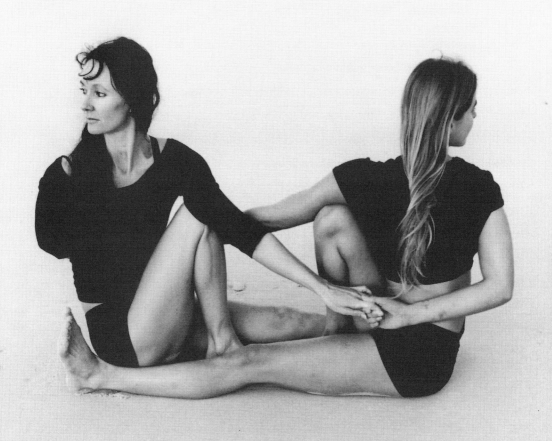

Ardha matsyendrasana release

ARDHA—HALF; MATSYENDRA—LORD OF THE FISHES

In the posture: One partner sits with their legs outstretched. Bend your left leg, placing the foot beside your right hip, knee to the floor. Step your right foot over your left leg, placing it on the outside of your left knee. Inhale to lift, thinning your waist, and exhale to turn to look over your right shoulder. Place your right hand on the floor behind your right hip and bend your left arm, locking the elbow in front of your right knee.

Adjuster: Sit behind your partner, place your right hand on their right shoulder and your left hand on their waist above their left hip. As they inhale to lift, lift their torso; as they exhale to twist, assist the rotation by turning their right shoulder out and rotating their left waist toward the front.

Breathe: Inhale to lift, exhale to twist.

Focus: Release tension and tightness in the spine.

Hold: 5–10 deep, full breaths, then release and twist to the other side. Then swap positions with your partner.

Benefits: Stretches and tones the spinal cord; massages and cleanses the internal organs; relieves a sore back and releases tension in the spine; stimulates the metabolism and refreshes the brain.

A stimulating twist for developing our sense of balance and coordination.

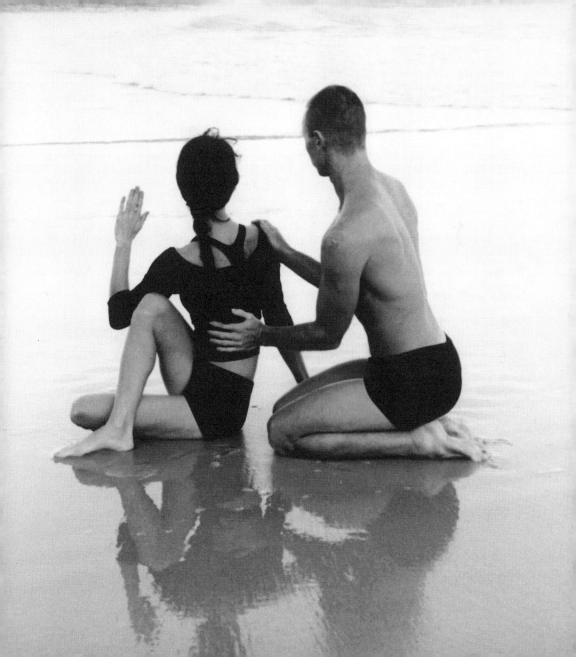

Invigorating and refreshing, backward-bending postures turn the body inside out, challenging its flexibility. With regular practice, stiffness is replaced with suppleness, and physical limitations are overcome by litheness and limberness. Tight chest and back muscles and shoulders are nourished with fresh blood, increasing elasticity and durability.

A strong back is fundamental to our health. As the keystone of our physical body, a supple, flexible toned back is integral to our well-being. The spinal nerves, which feed the organs of our entire body, are toned and strengthened along with the muscles of the whole back. Tension and wastes are washed away and replaced with a softness and mobility that reflect youth and agility.

Backbends are a powerful antidote to depression. When you open the chest, heart and lungs, built-up negative emotions are released and the brain is regenerated with a fresh supply of nutritious blood and oxygen, attributing to lively clear-headedness and positive mental and emotional states.

Be with your partner in an open-hearted space, inspiring love in each other.

Breathe in unison and communicate clearly about the adjustments to avoid injury. Warm up before practicing to avoid straining. Rest between backbending postures to prevent dizziness, and rest in a forward stretch to counterbalance the flexion. Avoid backward-bending positions if you have high blood pressure, a weak heart, a back injury or are pregnant.

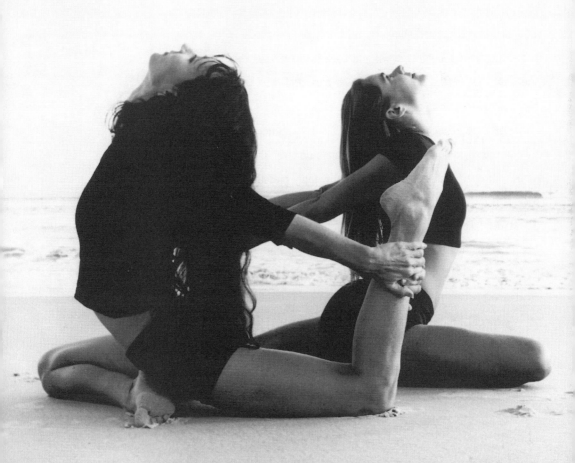

Backward-bending boosters

Urdhva mukha svanasana opening

URDHVA–UP; MUKHA–FACE; SVANA–DOG

In the posture: One partner lies on their stomach, legs extending away, arms bent and palms to the floor beside their shoulders. Inhale and lift your head, chest and shoulders off the floor, straightening your arms and rolling your shoulders down and back to open your chest. Squeeze your buttocks, extend out of your lower back and drop your head back and look toward the tip of your nose.

Adjuster: Stand behind your partner, bend your knees and place one knee into their middle back with your hands on their shoulders. As they exhale, roll their shoulders back and gently apply pressure to the middle back, moving it in and up to encourage a deeper opening in the chest.

Breathe: Take deep, full breaths through the nose.

Focus: Lengthen out of the lower back, open the chest and extend the legs away.

Hold: 5–10 deep, full breaths, then release, rest and swap positions with your partner.

Variation: Stay looking forward if it strains your neck to look back.

Benefits: Opens the chest cavity, respiratory muscles, heart, lungs and throat; promotes deep, full breathing; strengthens the back.

Rolling up and out, open your heart to the delicious lightness of being.

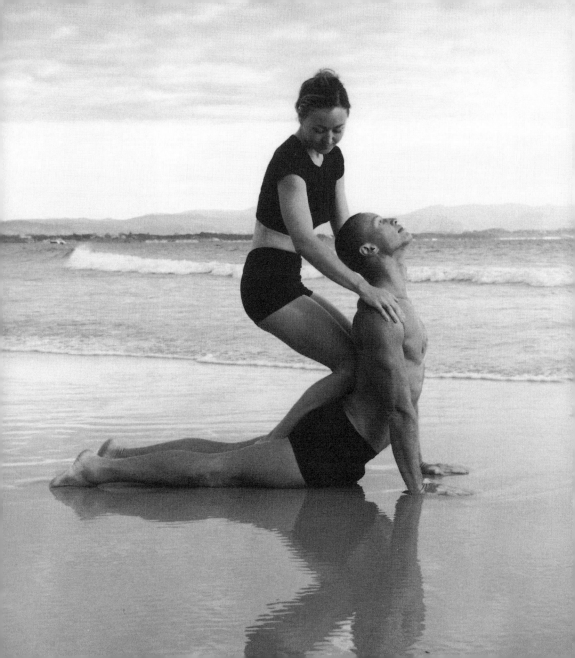

Salabhasana lift

SALABHA—LOCUST

In the posture: One partner lies on their stomach, legs extending away, forehead to the floor. Inhale to lift your head, chest, shoulders and arms off the ground. Extend your arms away, palms facing each other. Squeeze your buttocks and lift your chest higher. Focus on a point at eye level ahead.

Adjuster: Stand behind your partner with your feet on either side of their legs. Bend your knees and hold their wrists. As they exhale and soften, draw their arms back to encourage more lift and opening in their chest.

Breathe: Take deep, full breaths, focusing on softening on the exhalation.

Focus: Soften in the back and open the chest.

Hold: 5–10 breaths, then release, rest and swap positions with your partner.

Benefits: Strengthens the back muscles and tones the spinal nerves; opens and strengthens the chest muscles; promotes deep, full breathing; massages and cleanses the abdominal organs, kidney, liver and intestines; aids in relieving stomach disorders.

With the hips dropping into the ground, rest freely into this supported body lift.

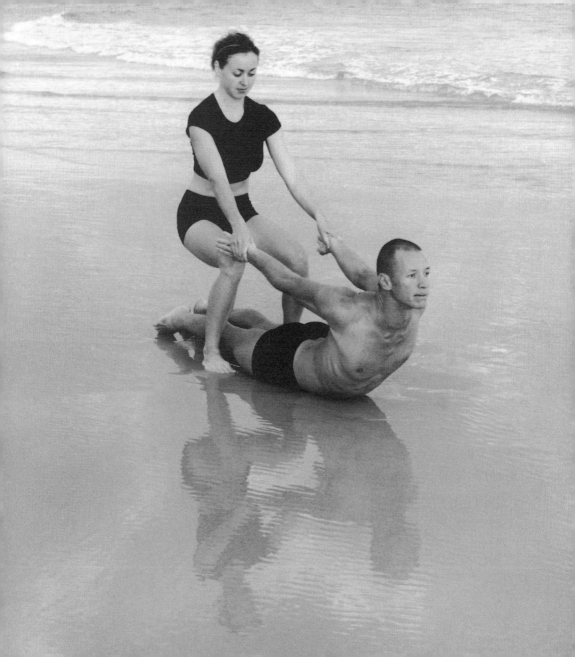

Purvottanasana lift

PURVA—EAST

In the posture: One partner sits legs outstretched, feet together and palms on the ground behind their hips, fingers facing forward. Take a deep breath in, puffing your chest out with air. On the exhale, lift your hips and buttocks off the floor, lock your legs and arms, and drop your head back. Press your toes into the floor, squeeze your buttocks and lift your hips higher. Focus on the tip of your nose.

Adjuster: When they have lifted their body fully, stand over your partner, feet either side of their knees, and position your hands under their hips. Assist them with the upward lift, keeping your knees bent.

Breathe: Inhale deeply, filling your chest, and lift higher with each full exhalation.

Focus: Keep your toes to the floor, squeeze your buttocks and elevate your hips.

Hold: 5–10 breaths, then release, rest and swap positions with your partner.

Benefits: Stretches the entire front of the body; opens the chest, heart and lungs, and promotes deep, full breathing; strengthens the legs, feet and ankles; opens the throat.

Elevating to new heights, stretch open your heart and throat for clear communication.

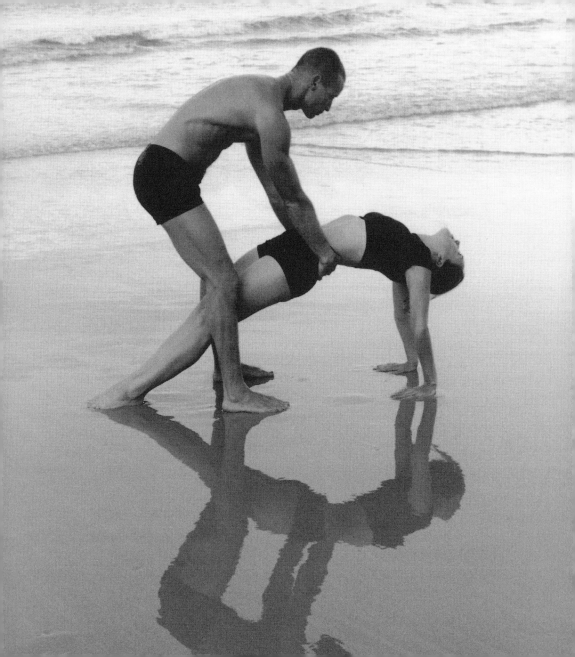

Mini backbend lift

In the posture: One partner lies on their back, feet hip-width apart beside their buttocks. Place your arms by your side, palms facing down. Raise your buttocks and hips, arching your back and pressing your feet into the floor. Work your knees towards each other so your legs are parallel. Feel the support coming from your feet, arms, neck and shoulders. Maintain a soft eye gaze to your navel.

Adjuster: Kneel beside your partner. When they have lifted their body fully, position your hands under their hips and assist them with the upward lift.

Breathe: Inhale deeply and fully to fill your chest, exhale fully to lift higher.

Focus: Keep your toes to the floor, squeeze your buttocks and keep your knees aligned with the hips.

Hold: 5–10 breaths, then release down, rest, and change positions.

Benefits: Stretches and massages the abdominal organs; helps correct rounded shoulders and poor posture; tones the sexual organs; tones the muscles of the entire front of the body; strengthens the legs and feet.

Feel the skin on your abdomen stretch over your belly as your hips lift higher and higher.

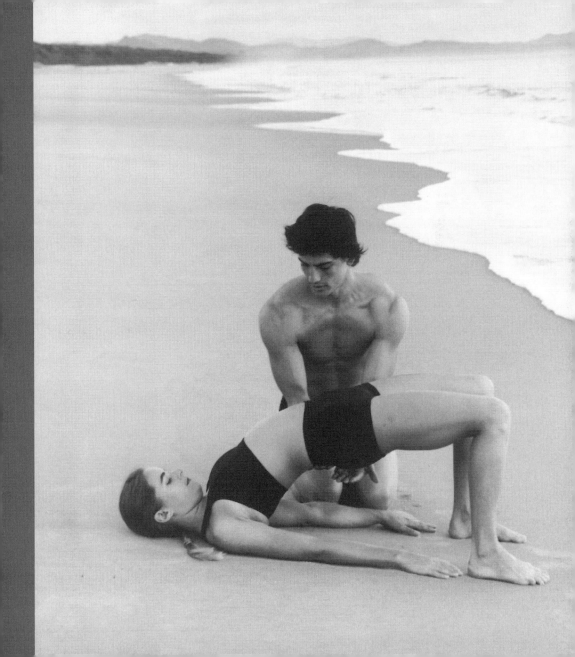

Urdhva dhanurasana supported lift

URDHVA–UPWARDS; DHANURA–BOW

In the posture: One partner lies on the floor, the soles of their feet hip-width apart beside their buttocks. Hold the front of your partner's ankles above your head. On the inhalation, push your feet into the floor, activating your inner leg muscles and pressing into your partner's ankles; lift your buttocks and hips off the floor, and rest the top of your head on the floor. On the next inhalation breath, straighten your arms by pushing into your partner's ankles, lift your chest and hips high, and drop your head back to look at the floor.

Adjuster: Once your partner has hold of your ankles, bend forward to wrap your hands around the sides of their torso. As they inhale and lift, draw them up towards you. Once they are fully lifted, move their chest closer towards you with your hands under their chest.

Breathe: Take deep, full breaths, open your chest.

Focus: Balance your body weight evenly between your feet and hands. Lift and lengthen out of your lower back.

Hold: 5–10 deep, full breaths, then release down.

Benefits: Stretches the back and abdominal muscles; massages the abdominal organs, and stimulates digestion and the metabolism; increases blood supply to the brain.

Slowly **rise** to full flexion, one step at a **time**, with the **breath** as a guide and your partner for **support**.

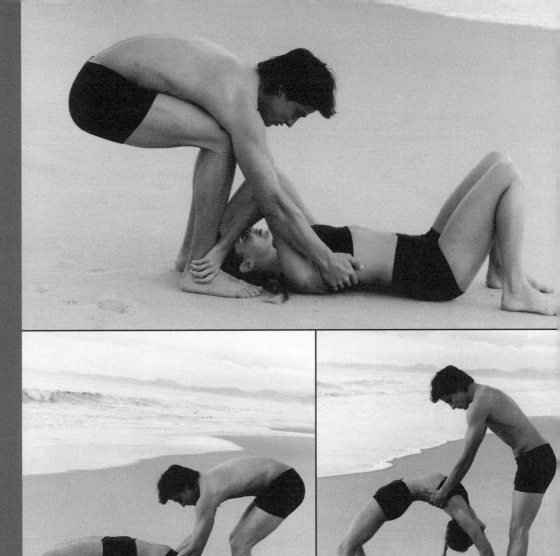

Dhanurasana elevation

DHANURA–BOW

In the posture: One partner lies flat on their stomach, forehead to the floor. Bend your knees, drawing your feet towards your head. Hold your ankles and squeeze your buttocks as you lift your thighs and feet upwards, and head and chest off the floor. Look forward and focus on balancing on your stomach and the front of your hips.

Adjuster: Stand behind and over your partner, bending your knees to support your own back as you lift. When your partner is fully lifted, hold their wrists and pull them upwards, encouraging a deeper lift and back flexion. Experiment with the adjustment. If you pull their hands towards you, their chest lifts higher off the ground; if you lift their hands and feet upwards, their legs lift higher off the ground. Aim for a centered lift.

Breathe: Inhale to lift, exhale to soften and relax in the pose.

Focus: Press your lower back downward; lift your chest; pull your feet toward you with your arms.

Hold: 5–10 breaths, or for as long as is comfortable, then release down, rest and change positions with your partner.

Benefits: Opens the shoulders; tones and strengthens the back and spinal cord; tones the entire back of the body.

A gorgeous arch to tone and stimulate the whole back, increasing flexibility and vitality.

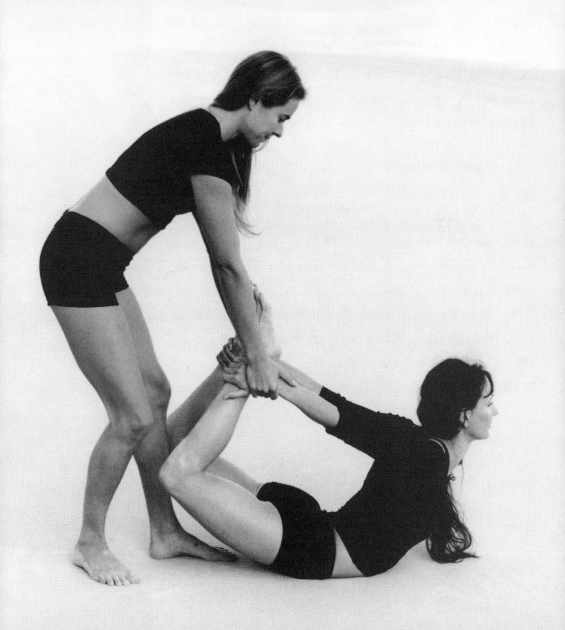

Back arch

In the posture: Stand back to back with your partner about a yard apart. Have your feet together and activate your legs, drawing your kneecaps and thighs upwards. Inhale to lift out of your waist, extending your arms upwards. As you lift, tuck your tailbone under and extend out of your lower back, feeling the vertebrae elongate and separate. Extend your arms back behind your head and join hands with your partner.

Breathe: As you exhale, soften in your back; as you inhale, lift and expand your chest.

Focus: Soften into the back arch with the breath, keeping your legs locked.

Hold: 3–5 breaths, then release slowly with the out breath. If you cannot reach your partner's hands, step closer together.

Benefits: Tones the back muscles and spinal cord; stimulates circulation throughout the spine and entire body; expands the chest, heart and lungs.

Like a green branch bending back in the wind, find each other in an invigorating bend.

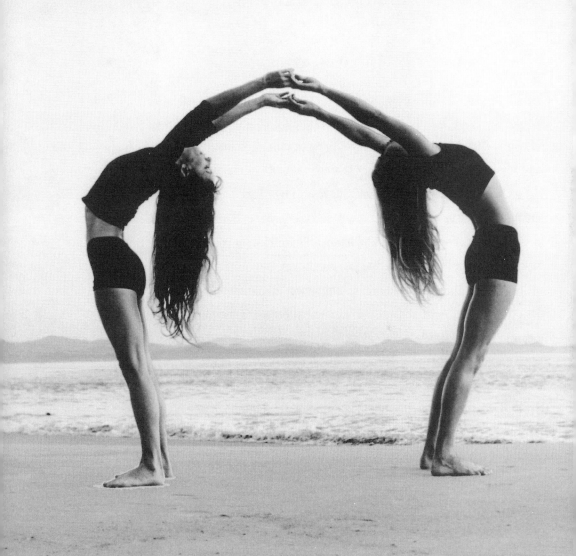

Virabhadrasana I
back arch

VIRA—WARRIOR FROM INDIAN MYTHOLOGY

In the posture: Both partners perform the posture with their right leg forward first. Stand back to back about a yard apart. Step your right foot forward and lunge down into your right leg to create a right angle, your knee above your ankle. Turn your back foot out 45° and lock the back leg. Join the outside edge of your left foot with your partner's and press them into the floor. Rotate your left hip forward, and your right hip back. Inhale to lift out of your waist and raise your arms. Exhale to drop your arms back, lift out of your lower back and join hands with your partner above and behind you. Drop your head back to look at your hands.

Breathe: Inhale to lift and expand your chest, exhale to soften and release in your back.

Focus: Keep your back foot pressing into your partner's. Lift out of your waist and keep your right leg at a right angle, the knee above the ankle.

Hold: 5–10 deep, full breaths, then release and repeat on the other side.

Benefits: Stimulates the nervous system; tones the spinal cord; softens the back muscles; opens the shoulders and strengthens the legs and knee joints.

A dynamic and stimulating pose for developing inner strength and willpower.

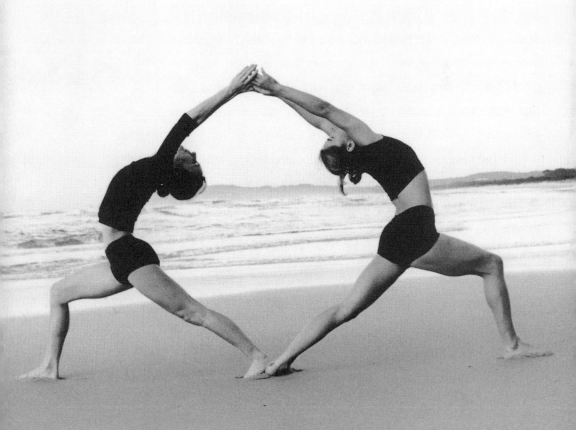

Lunging forward, reaching back

In the posture: Stand back to back with your partner about one to two yards apart. Lunge down into your right knee, your left leg extending back with the knee resting on the floor and toes turned under. Lunge forward, then inhale to lift out of your waist and raise your arms. Exhale to drop your head back and reach over with your arms to hold your partner's hands. Keep lifting out of your waist and lengthening out of your lower back as you arch backwards. Maintain soft eye focus up to your hands.

Breathe: Lift and expand your chest fully with the breath.

Focus: Drop your hips, lift your torso, soften your back.

Hold: 5 breaths, or for as long as is comfortable.

Variation: Position yourselves closer together for a less intense back arch.

Benefits: Opens the chest, heart, lungs and shoulders; stretches the back and pelvic muscles; stimulates the nervous system.

As the chest lifts and expands and the back arches, feel the kidneys being toned and the whole body being washed with stimulating heat.

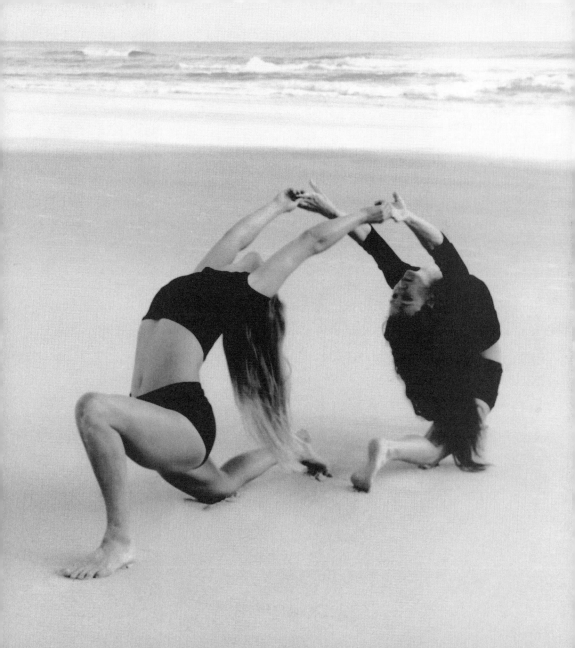

Ustrasana wrap

USTRA—CAMEL

In the posture: Kneel facing your partner about a yard apart, your knees and feet hip-width apart. Hold each other's arms and inhale to lift out of your waist. On the exhalation, slowly drop your head back and come into a back arch. Using each other for support, drop further into the back arch with each exhalation. Keep your hips in line with your knees.

Breathe: Soften into your back with the exhalation breath; lift out of your lower back with the inhalation breath.

Focus: Lengthen out of your lower back.

Hold: 5–10 breaths, or for as long as is comfortable, then release and rest in a forward stretch to counter-balance the backbend.

Benefits: Opens the chest, heart and lungs, and stretches the respiratory muscles; flexes the back and encourages a healthy, supple spine.

Find beauty and grace in a harmonious practice that mirrors your two souls in peace.

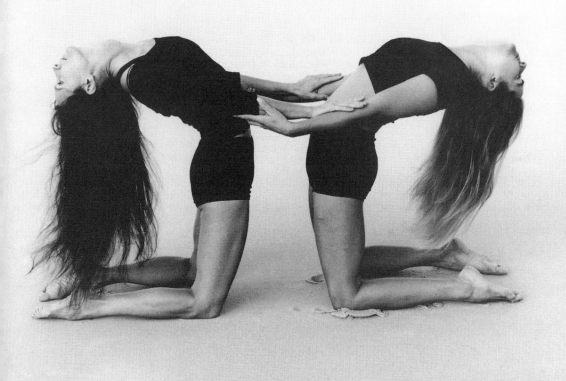

Ustrasana doubles

USTRA—CAMEL

In the posture: Kneel facing your partner, your feet and knees hip-width apart. Be hip to hip with your partner so that your pubis bones are touching. Moving together, inhale to lift out of your waist. Exhale to drop your head back, and slowly release your palms down one at a time to rest on the soles of your feet. Lift out of your lower back and lengthen your spine upwards to open your chest out. Breathe into the upper chest. Be centered with your partner, creating one straight line from your hips to your knees. To release up, inhale to lift the head, then allow the arms to come up.

Breathe: Maintain deep, full breaths.

Focus: Lift out of your lower back so there is no compression. If your back feels sore, release out slowly with the breath and counterbalance the pose by resting in a forward-bending posture or Lengthening Forward (page 188).

Hold: 5–10 deep, full breaths, then release and rest in a forward stretch to counter-pose the backbend.

Benefits: Opens the chest and shoulders; stretches the stomach and intestines, helping to relieve intestinal disorders; relieves backache and promotes good posture.

Softness, mobility and lightness are created within these beautiful curves.

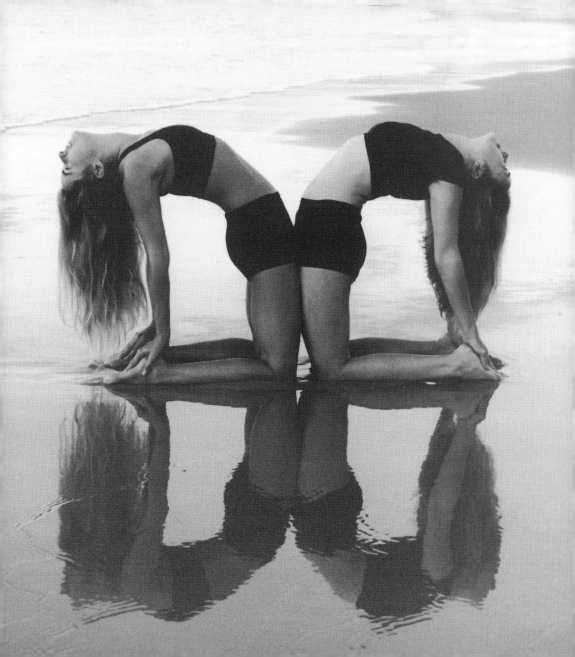

Ustrasana cupped

USTRA–CAMEL

In the posture: Performed simultaneously, one partner comes into the full *Ustrasana* position (on previous page) while the other person rests in a supported variation of *Ustrasana* on their partner. The partner practicing the full pose kneels with their feet and knees hip-width apart. Inhale to lift out of your waist and exhale to drop your head back and slowly place the palms of your hands onto the soles of your feet one at a time. Lifting out of your lower back, breathe fully up into your chest and move your pubis forward. The other partner kneels with their feet on the outside of their partner's legs. Inhale to lift out of your waist, exhale to drop your head back and move your pubis forward. Rest the back of your head on your partner's chest. Rest your arms by your side to hold your partner's legs.

Breathe: Inhale fully up into your chest.

Focus: Keep your gaze towards the tip of your nose.

Hold: 5–10 deep, full breaths, then the top partner inhales up to release first. Rest and change positions.

Benefits: Opens the chest and shoulders; stretches the stomach and intestines, helping to relieve intestinal disorders; relieves backache and promotes good posture.

A loving embrace to relax in the openness of each other's heart and feel supported in rest.

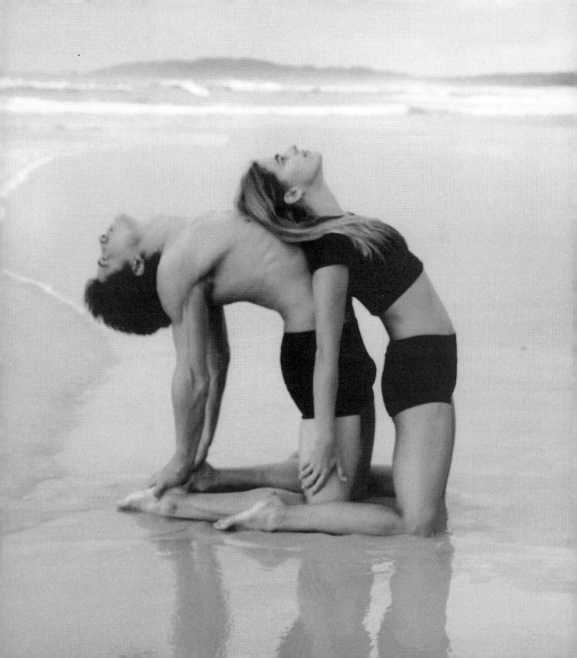

Kapotasana doubles

KAPOTA–PIGEON

In the posture: One person comes into the full posture, which is the more intense back arch, while the second person rests on the top in the easy variation. Kneel back to back with your partner, your feet and knees hip-width apart and the tips of your toes touching your partner's. First person: inhale to lift out of your lower back and exhale to drop your head back and release your arms over your head to rest your hands on your partner's feet or legs (whichever you can reach). Second person: inhale and then exhale to drop back and rest your hands on your partner's torso (wherever is comfortable). Both partners should have a soft eye gaze to their third eye.

Breathe: Inhale to lift out of your lower back; exhale to soften and arch further back.

Focus: Keep your hips above your knees, lift and puff your chest outward.

Hold: 5–10 breaths, or for as long as is comfortable, then release up and rest in a forward stretch to counter-pose the backbend before changing positions.

Benefits: Tones the spinal muscles and spinal cord; promotes a healthy, supple back; opens the chest, heart and lungs; stimulates blood flow to the pelvic region.

The whole front of the body rounds outward in this intense backward arch.

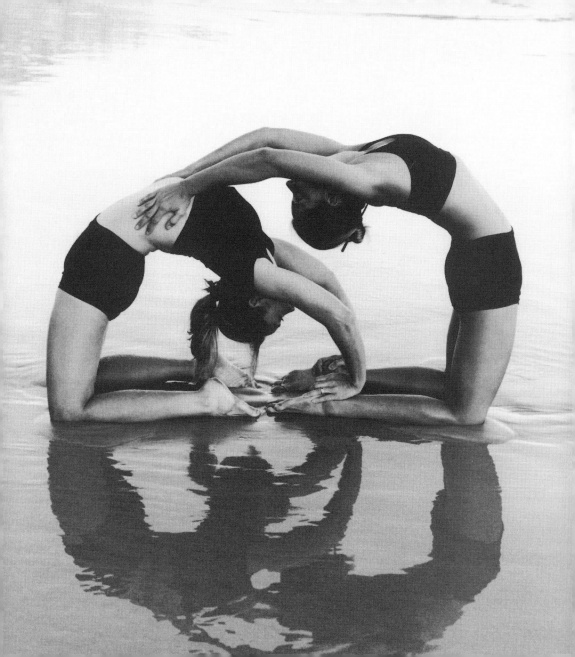

Rajakapotasana joining

RAJA–KING: KAPOTA–PIGEON

In the posture: Sit back to back with your partner, about a yard apart. Turn your right foot in to rest at the front of your left hip. Extend your left leg back behind you. Rotate the front of the left hip down to the ground so that both hips are parallel to the front. On the inhale, lift out of your waist, on the exhale bend your left leg and bring your arms back behind you one at a time to hold your partner's ankle with your right hand and your own ankle with your left hand. Stay looking forward, lifting out of your lower back and lifting and opening your chest.

Breathe: Take deep, full breaths.

Focus: Lift your chest; lift out of your lower back.

Hold: 5–10 breaths, then release and change sides.

Variation: If you have the opening, drop your head back and focus on the tip of your nose.

Benefits: Tones the back and spinal cord; stimulates blood flow to the pelvic and reproductive organs; opens the chest, heart and lungs.

A beautiful posture to share with a friend: the heart is open, the back is soft and the mind relaxed as the focus is turned inward.

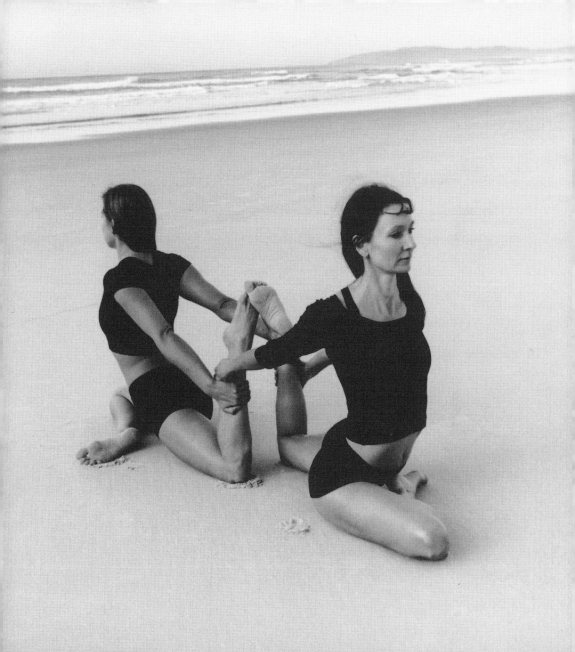

The healing powers of inversions are immense. We only need a few minutes upside down to reap the invigorating rewards—the supply of oxygen-rich blood increases to the spinal nerves and the entire body, re-energizing sluggish function and helping to combat disease and illness. The blood supply to the brain also increases, resulting in better concentration, mental focus and clarity.

Regularly positioning oneself upside down defies gravity and the aging process. When the head is positioned below the heart, the heart can redirect its energy, pumping enriching blood to the other body systems. The overall effect is an increase in circulation, the removal of wastes and the oxygenation of often underused parts of our anatomy, which all results in our feeling more energized and vital, and looking more vibrant and youthful.

The lungs also function well upside down, which results in deeper, fuller breathing. Deep breathing calms the nervous system, aids the release of stress and tension from the body and mind and helps to overcome anxiety.

The following simple postures will prepare your body for other more advanced, full-body inversions. It is easy to assist your partner in receiving the immense therapeutic benefits of these inversions with simple weightbearing and lifting adjustments. Practice together and experiment with your adjustments for best results.

Inversions are often beneficial for people with low blood pressure, but should be avoided by those with high blood pressure or a weak heart.

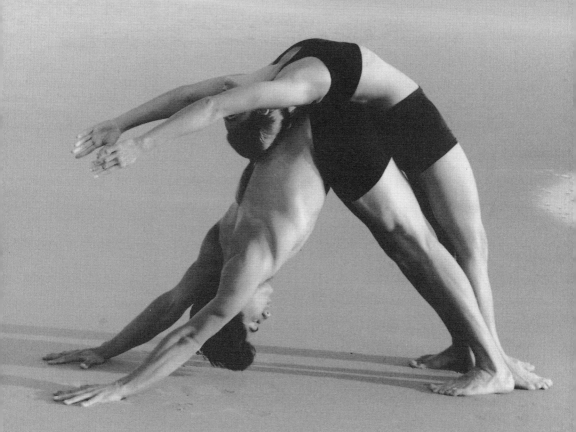

Inverting for health

Adho mukha svanasana lift

ADHO-DOWN; MUKHA-FACE; SVANA-DOG

In the posture: One partner kneels on the floor and extends forward. Stretch your arms and spread your fingers wide, your middle finger pointing forward. Step your right foot back, then your left. Straighten your legs, your feet hip-width apart, heels to the ground. Inhale and raise your buttocks and hips high; extend your spine upward. Lower the crown of your head downward. Relax your chest through your shoulders.

Adjuster: Sit on the ground between your partner's outstretched hands. Place your hands behind you and lean back into them for support as you adjust. Bend your knees and place your heels into your partner's shoulders. Lift their shoulders upwards, assisting the lift of their spine, hips and buttocks. Keep your back straight as you adjust, drawing your lower back in so it does not collapse.

Breathe: Inhale and exhale deeply and fully through the nose.

Focus: Extend your spine upwards; lift your hips and buttocks high and soften your head, neck and shoulders.

Hold: 10 deep, full breaths, then release, rest and swap positions.

Benefits: Elongates the spine; supplies the spinal nerves with oxygenated blood; stretches the hamstring muscles, and the muscles of the legs and arms; stimulates the flow of oxygenated blood to the brain.

Find equilibrium as your head and heart rest upside down.

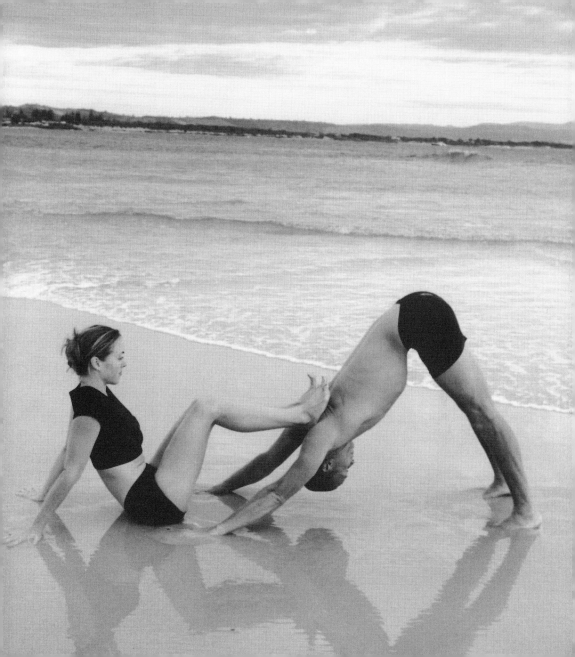

Adho mukha svanasana elongation

ADHO—DOWN; MUKHA—FACE; SVANA—DOG

In the posture: One partner kneels on the floor and extends forward. Stretch your arms and spread your fingers wide, your middle finger pointing forward. Step your right foot back, then your left. Straighten your legs, your feet hip-width apart. Inhale and raise your buttocks and hips high, extending your spine upward. Lower the crown of your head. Lift your shoulders up and away from your ears. Relax your chest through your shoulders and work your heels to the floor.

Adjuster: Stand between your partner's hands. Step one foot forward, bending the knee for support, and place the palms of your hands on your partner's sacral area. Lengthen their back by moving their sacrum upward. The aim is to elongate their spine upward.

Breathe: Inhale and exhale deeply into the chest.

Focus: Lengthen the spine; keep the buttocks and hips lifting upwards.

Hold: 10 deep, full breaths, then release, rest and swap positions.

Benefits: Lengthens the spine; separates the vertebrae; encourages circulation to the organs; stretches the hamstring muscles; stimulates circulation to the head and brain; refreshes the brain; cleanses the internal organs; stimulates the metabolism; strengthens the legs and arms.

Lengthen beyond your limitations with your partner's lift.

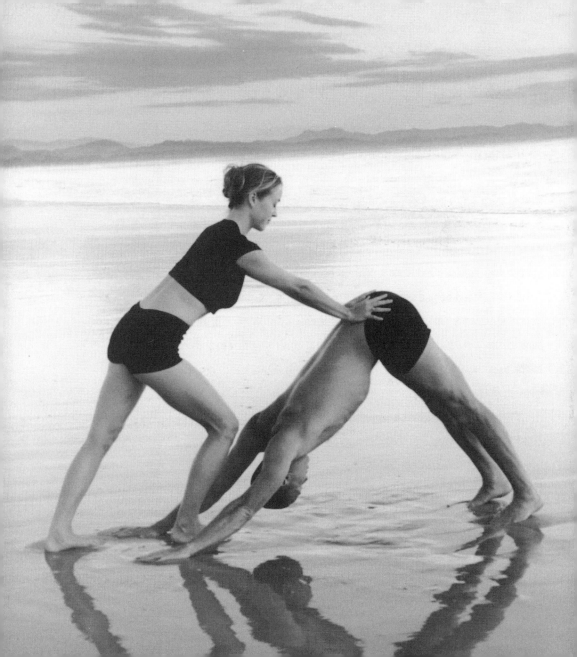

Adho mukha svanasana stretch

ADHO—DOWN; MUKHA—FACE; SVANA—DOG

In the posture: One partner kneels on the floor and extends forward. Stretch your arms and spread your fingers wide, your middle finger pointing forward. Step your right foot back, then your left. Straighten your legs, your feet hip-width apart. Inhale and raise your buttocks and hips high; extend your spine upward. Lower the crown of your head downward. Relax your chest through your shoulders and work your heels to the floor.

Adjuster: Stand behind your partner. Position your toes so that they are clenching your partner's heels and pressing them down. With your knees bent to support your back, hold your partner's upper thighs. Draw their thighs back toward you. This will encourage them to activate and lift their kneecaps and thigh muscles.

Breathe: Inhale and exhale evenly through your nose.

Focus: Keep your legs locked; extend your hips and buttocks upwards; lengthen your spine upwards.

Hold: 10 deep, full breaths, then release, rest, and swap positions.

Benefits: Stretches the hamstring and calf muscles and Achilles tendon; tones the sciatic nerve; stimulates circulation to the head and brain; cleanses the internal organs; stimulates the metabolism; strengthens the legs and arms.

Distribute your body weight evenly between your hands and feet to develop a sense of balance.

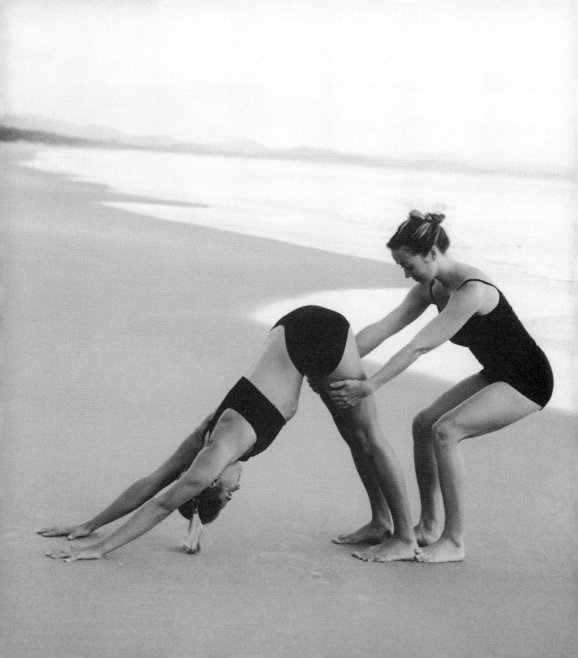

Upside down and dynamic

In the posture: One partner goes into the *Adho Mukha Svanasana* position as on the previous page.

Adjuster: In this inverted posture, you will be balancing on your partner's sacrum to apply a gentle lift. It is as much a doubles posture as an adjustment, so enjoy each other in strength and coordination! To come into the pose, sit in front of your partner in a squatting position until they are in position. Place your hands flat on the floor and when your partner is ready, raise one leg at a time and rest the balls of your feet on their sacral area. Lock your legs and roll your shoulders out, then lock your elbows and lift upward to create a 90° angle with your torso and legs. Lightly move your feet upward to lengthen your partner's spine.

Breathe: Inhale and exhale evenly for balance and steadiness in the postures.

Focus: Maintain balance and keep your legs and arms locked.

Hold: 10 breaths, or for as long as is comfortable for both partners. Then swap positions.

Benefits: Elongates the spine; stretches the hamstring muscles; tones the legs and arms; stimulates the flow of oxygenated blood to the brain; restorative effect on the heart.

Experiment with varying degrees of inversion and develop confidence as you play with upside-down postures.

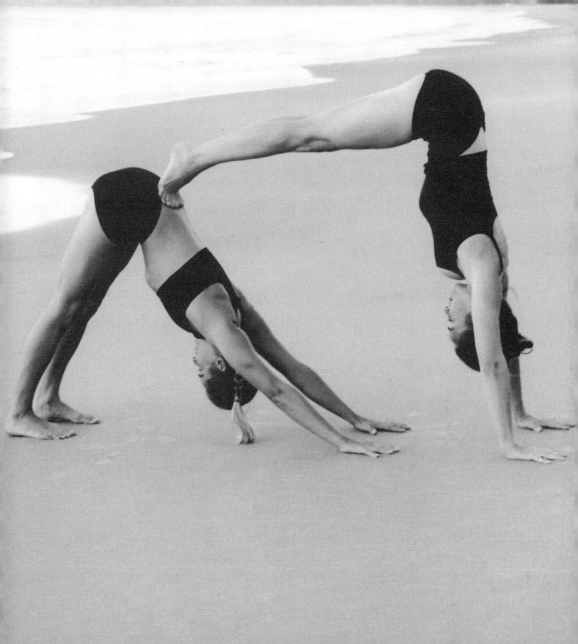

Taking the time out of a busy schedule to relax will restore your body's energy levels, refresh your mind and allow for a new lease on life. When highly stressed, the more we stop and relax, the more juice we'll have to deal with problems and approach life with focus and clarity.

Drawing our attention to tense areas and learning to relax them allows us to soften and rest the whole body, from the skin to the muscles and from the organs to the bones and joints. It is often not until we have applied ourselves consciously to the art of relaxation that we realize how much tension we hold on to.

When intending to relax completely, use the breath to soften and release tightness; feel it melting away with each deep, full breath. Bring your intention first to the most obviously tense areas, relax them, then move to subtler levels in the body and mind.

When beginning to relax, ask yourself what your intention is. Remind yourself that what you want from the practice is to feel completely relaxed, rejuvenated and calm, then lie back and let your body and mind release, ahhh . . .

Enjoy some time in a relaxation pose between other postures, and rest in *Savasana* for at least 5–10 minutes at the end of a yoga practice to restore the body and mind to calm.

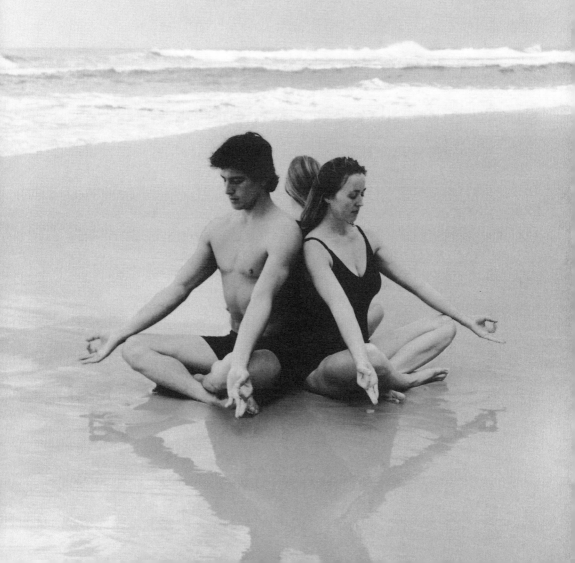

Real calm

Savasana

SAVA—LIFELESS BODY

In the posture: Lie on your back beside your partner. Make the space between you small so you are aware of each other's presence. Let your feet and legs fall away from each other. Rest your arms beside your body, palms facing upwards. Tuck your chin in and extend the back of your neck on the floor. Have the lips slightly parted. Adjust your body so it feels comfortable. Close your eyes. Find any areas of your body that are holding tension and relax them completely.

Breathe: Inhale and exhale slowly, softly, naturally.

Focus: Observe your breath. Whenever you find yourself thinking, return your awareness to your breath. Relax the muscles of your whole body, from the muscles of your scalp and the skin on your face, down to your toes. Sink deeper and deeper into relaxation.

Hold: 10 minutes, or longer at the end of your yoga session. Practice for a few breaths when you need a rest, especially after dynamic postures. To release, roll to your right side and slowly come up to sitting.

Variation: Cover your eyes with an eye bag or cloth to relax your eye muscles and help relieve a headache.

Benefits: Relaxes the entire body; rests the nervous system and quiets the mind; develops concentration and self-awareness; practiced before sleeping, helps relieve insomnia.

Bathe in the stillness and quiet of non-thinking and non-doing.

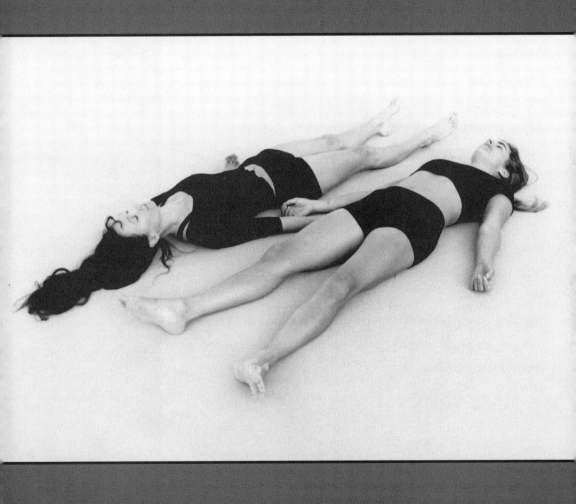

Inward bound

In the posture: One partner sits with their buttocks on their heels. Lean forward and rest your torso on your knees, and the backs of your arms on the floor alongside your legs, the palms facing upward. Rest your forehead on the floor, drop your shoulders and relax every muscle in your body. Feel your head and body sinking into deep relaxation.

Adjuster: Stand at your partner's side, bending forward with your knees bent and apply pressure to their back, gently pressing their lower back down and the upper back forward. This adjustment lengthens the spine and softens the back.

Breathe: Inhale and exhale slowly and naturally.

Focus: Close your eyes and let your body sink into the floor.

Hold: For as long as required to calm your mind and restore your energy levels.

Benefits: Calms the mind; slows the nervous system, heart rate and breathing; a soothing pose for resting in-between postures or whenever you need to relax.

Journey within to find yourself nurtured, warm and secluded in your center.

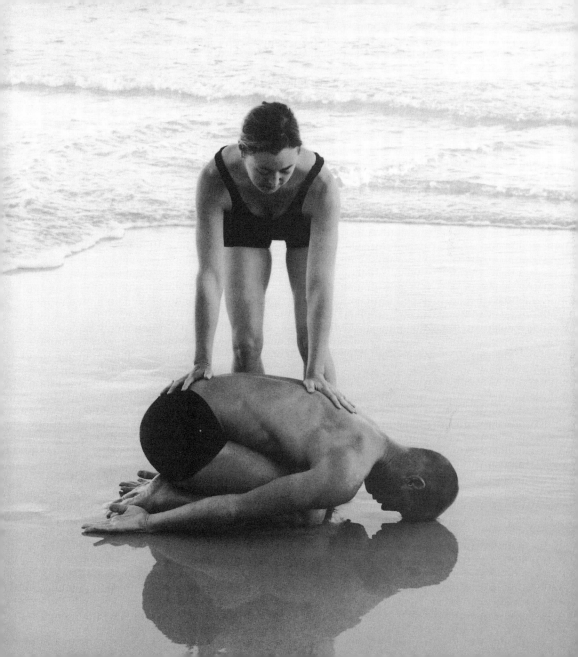

Lengthening forward

In the posture: One partner kneels on the floor, their big toes together and knees apart. Sit your buttocks back between your heels, onto the soles of your feet. Cup your fingers onto the floor in front of you. Inhale to lengthen out of your hips. Exhale and slowly release forward and down, walking your arms forward as you extend and rest your forehead on the floor. Keep your buttocks back on your heels and stretch your arms forward.

Adjuster: Stand beside and over your partner with your knees bent. Apply gentle pressure to their lower and upper back, lengthening their spine in two directions: the lower back moving back towards the buttocks and the upper back moving forward towards the arms.

Breathe: Inhale and exhale evenly through the nose.

Focus: Keep your buttocks down to the floor; elongate your spine.

Hold: 10 breaths, or for as long as required to lengthen the back. Practice after a backbend to release the muscles.

Benefits: Elongates the spine; separates the vertebrae; increases circulation and nerve supply to the organs of the body; helps create a supple back; opens the hips and stretches the groin muscles.

Be in position to **elongate** your vertebrae for a healthy, **flexible** spine.

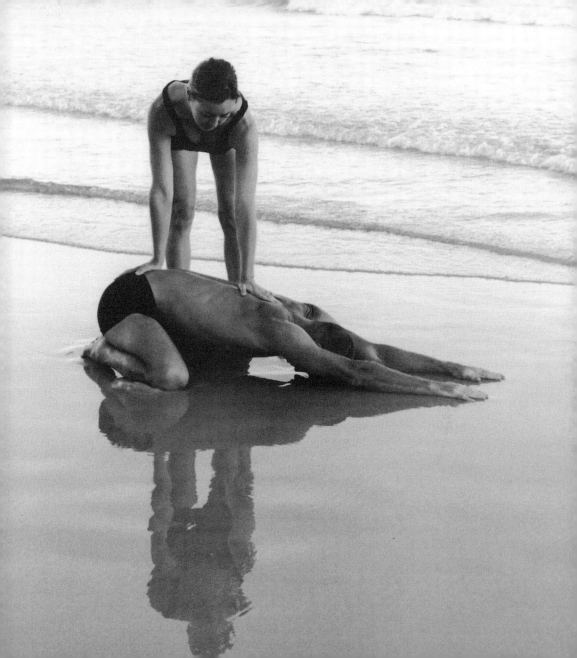

Kids love to move their bodies, explore their potential, create and connect with others and have fun. They are naturally present in the moment and open to learning and growing. Introducing your child to yoga at a young age has enormous benefits. Encouraging attributes of openness, flexibility, sharing and caring in young children promotes happy and healthy beings as well as a peaceful future.

Most of us are born naturally flexible and aligned, but as children we often mimic the posture of those around us and take on poor postural patterns. I have seen many extremely vibrant, fit and healthy five year olds who can no longer touch their toes. Regular stretching and breath awareness from a young age will set the foundation for a flexible body and a fluid life.

Experiment with your children in yoga postures and encourage them to practice together. As you watch their practice you'll soon discover their tight areas and weak points. Introduce them to postures that are effective in stretching tight areas and strengthening weak areas.

As well as physical benefits, yoga offers children access to increased mental focus, better balance and coordination, and more willpower and inner strength—all vital assets for growing. Set in a non-threatening and creative environment where they have the opportunity to be stimulated and creative, yoga for kids is fun for all.

The following postures offer inspiration for you and your children. Be creative, go with the flow and discover your child in yoga.

Kids' yoga

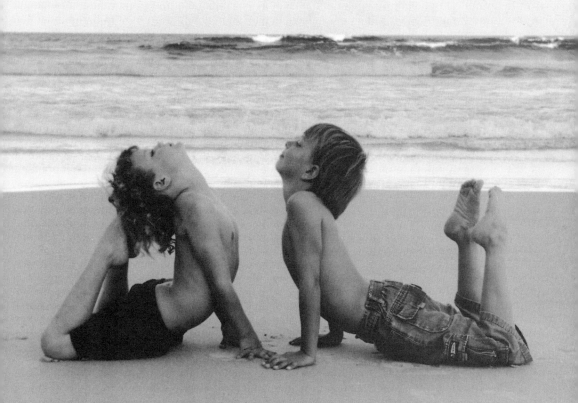

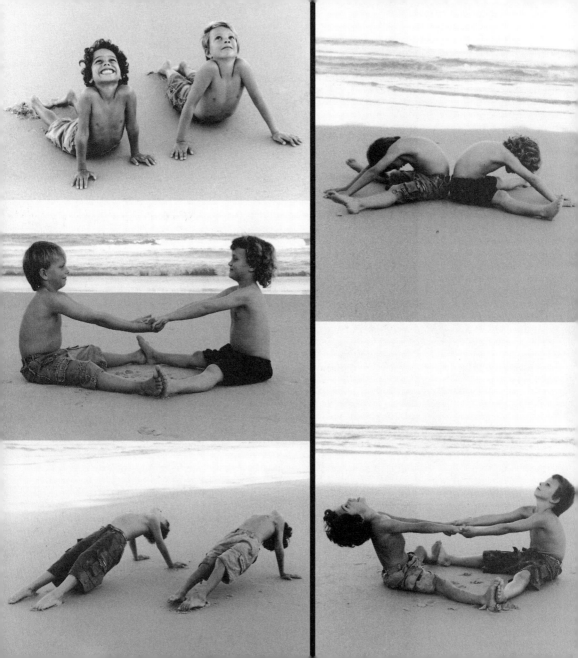

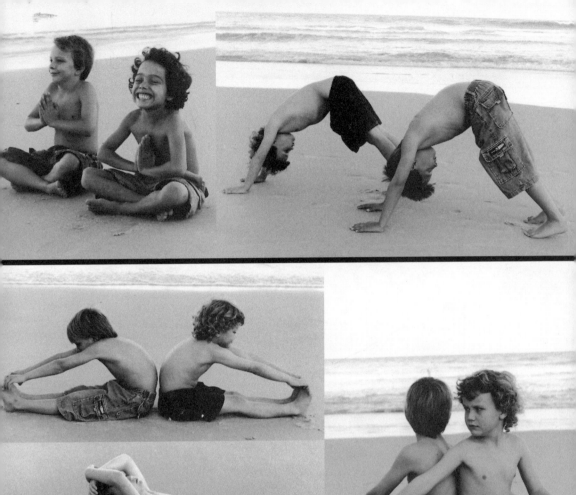
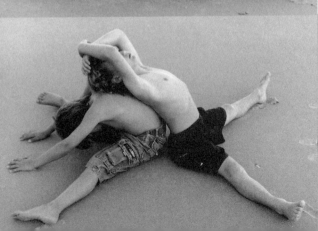
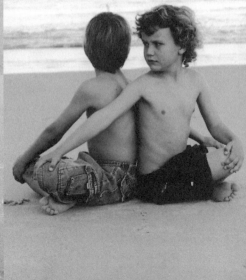

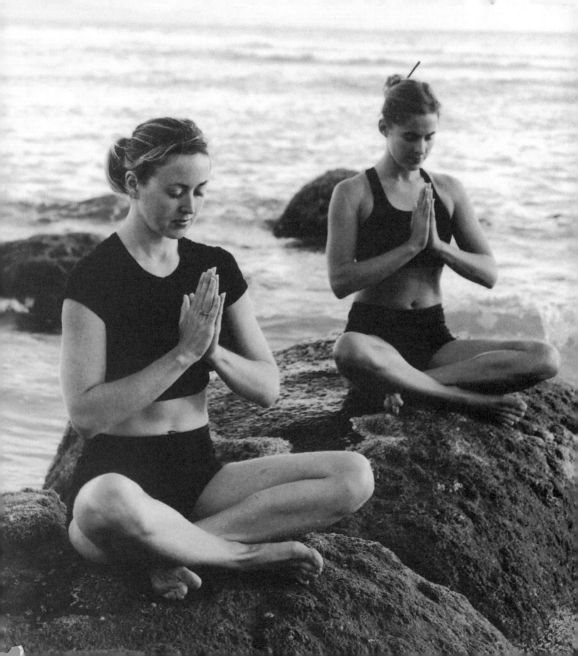